Stereoscopic manual of
the ocular fundus
in local and systemic disease

Stereoscopic manual of the ocular fundus in local and systemic disease

Frederick C. Blodi, M.D.

Associate Professor of Ophthalmology,
State University of Iowa College of Medicine,
Iowa City, Iowa

and

Lee Allen

Associate in Ophthalmology,
Iowa City, Iowa
State University of Iowa College of Medicine,

With a Foreword by

Alson E. Braley, M.D.

Head and Professor, Department of Ophthalmology, State University
of Iowa College of Medicine, Iowa City, Iowa

With 6 line drawings, 95 photomicrographs,
105 stereoscopic views in full color on 15 VIEW-MASTER®
reels, and a VIEW-MASTER® compact viewer

The C. V. Mosby Company   *Saint Louis*   *1964*

Foreword

The Department of Ophthalmology at the State University of Iowa College of Medicine has had a continuous tradition of fine medical art and photography. Dr. Cecil S. O'Brien, Professor and first Head of the Department, placed great importance upon good illustrations for classroom teaching, patients' records, and publications. The widely known ophthalmic artist, Mr. E. G. Bethke, now at The Institute of Ophthalmology, Columbia University College of Physicians and Surgeons, began his career at the State University of Iowa College of Medicine under the guidance of Dr. O'Brien. Emphasis was placed upon drawings of the fundus, and the Department still prizes the many fine color drawings done in those first years. Dr. A. R. Kahler, then a resident in ophthalmology and now in Sacramento, California, produced fine black and white photographs of the fundus with the encouragement of Dr. O'Brien. These were used to illustrate points of importance in diagnosis as well as for teaching aids.

For the past twenty-six years, our artist, Mr. Lee Allen, who also started in ophthalmic illustration under Dr. O'Brien and who was taught fundus drawing by his close friend, Mr. Bethke, has sustained the impetus for fine visual records and communications. He has always had the help and interest of both the teaching and resident staffs. One of the residents, Dr. N. Douvas, now in Dearborn, Michigan, began taking color transparency photographs with the Nordenson Retinal Camera soon after Dr. Arthur Bedell of Albany, New York, showed his first pictures taken on that film. The practical advantages of good color photography over time-consuming drawing of the fundus appealed to Mr. Allen, who immediately joined Dr. Douvas in perfecting a dependable photographic procedure. They were aided immeasurably in solving technical problems by personal communications from and encouragement by Dr. Bedell. Since that time, Mr. Allen has given a considerable amount of attention to making numerous good photographs of the fundus and to attempting to improve their quality and their value to the Department. There has been improvement with the advent of new, faster films and finer cameras and with the increased knowledge that comes from long experience.

Over the years, we have accumulated an enormous collection of single pictures of the fundus. This is undoubtedly true for Dr. Bedell and for institutions over the country. To our knowledge, only Dr. Bedell has presented an atlas from this huge body of material.

This Department was shown some of the excellent stereoscopic photographs of the fundus being done by Dr. Michael Hogan and Diane Beeston at the University of California. This stimulated Mr. Allen to employ this technique, to systematize it, and to make it the routine method for case records. Already, a very comprehensive collection of fundus pathology in stereoscopic view has been gathered. Selections from this collection make up the present graphic manual.

This publication is clearly an outgrowth of the early work in the Department in both drawing and photography plus all of the outside stimuli and help previously mentioned.

The stereoscopic effect observed in the reels can be said to be slightly exaggerated, especially by comparison with the photographs shown by Dr. Bedell, Dr. David Donaldson, and others. This exaggeration cannot be termed "false" any more than can magnification, and these two "tools" combined in the stereophotographs help in revealing relative depths of lesions even in such fine structures as the retina. Stereoscopic pictures in color have great value as a diagnostic tool. There is no doubt after seeing many such pictures that repeated examination will reveal new features and more detail than when looking at the fundus with the ophthalmoscope. Many times, with periodic, successive stereophotographs, the appearance or disappearance of opacities within the retina can be followed in detail. The progression or resolution of chorioretinal lesions may also be followed. Consequently, the stereoscopic pictures have an additional, definite value for following up lesions of the fundus.

Stereophotographs of the fundus have a tremendous potential for teaching. They might give medical students or neophytes in ophthalmology their first opportunity to see and clearly understand many details of both the normal and the abnormal fundus. If, later, they do not have stereoscopic views to aid them, the classroom presentation of stereophotographs might have amounted to their only opportunity to gain real insight into the meaning of the single two-dimensional ophthalmic views they will see in medical practice. Furthermore, these views and accompanying text can be an excellent "refresher" for the busy ophthalmologist.

Technical advances by Dr. Hans Littmann, who designed the modern Zeiss fundus camera, the creators of modern color film, and ingenuity of Mr. Lee Allen have made these stereoscopic pictures possible. In this book Dr. Frederick C. Blodi has collected the stereophotographs and the summaries of the cases, has included photomicrographs, and has written descriptive text material to explain the nature and locations of lesions.

In addition to its teaching value, this book will be helpful to practicing physicians in all fields of medicine in arriving at a correct diagnosis of lesions of the fundus through comparison of the fundi of their patients with the stereophotographs herein.

Alson E. Braley, M.D.

Preface

This book is an outgrowth of an exhibit presented at the American Medical Association in Atlantic City in June, 1963, and at the American Academy of Ophthalmology and Otolaryngology in New York in October, 1963. Many of the viewers expressed a desire to have a permanent collection of these pictures available. Since the value of the stereoscopic views in teaching and in diagnosis was pointed out, we thought it advisable also to include in the book illustrative photomicrographs which should help to clarify the nature and location of the various lesions.

Fundus pictures have been published ever since fundus photography was perfected. Dimmer and Pillat[*] and later Bedell[†] in this country have pioneered in this field. The most modern of reproductions[‡§‖] have improved in quality and added color as an essential attribute of these pictures.

Stereoscopic reproductions of the ocular fundus have been tried before.[¶‡] This has been done by drawings or by somewhat crude attempts of black and white photography. No stereoscopic manual has appeared during the last forty years.

Stereoscopic fundus pictures are being taken at other centers, notably at the University of California in San Francisco and at the Howe Laboratories of the Massachusetts Eye and Ear Infirmary. Both centers have influenced us, and the University of California in San Francisco has preceded us in taking such pictures.

There are some specific differences in the character of our pictures from most others we have seen. We purposely have not used the circular border masks

---

[*]Dimmer, J., and Pillat, A.: Atlas des Augenhintergrundes, Wien, 1927, F. Deuticke.
[†]Bedell, A. J.: Photographs of the fundus oculi, Philadelphia, 1929, F. A. Davis Co.
[‡]Ballantyne, A. J., and Michaelson, I. C.: Textbook of the fundus of the eye, Baltimore, 1963, Williams & Wilkins Co.
[§]Larsen, F.: Atlas of the fundus of the eye, Kopenhagen, 1963, E. Munksgaard.
[‖]Sautter, H., and Straub, W.: Der photographierte Augenhintergrund, München und Berlin, 1963, Urban und Schwarzenberg.
[¶]Bothman, L., and Bennett, R. W.: Fundus atlas, Chicago, 1939, Year Book Publishers, Inc.
[‡]Oatman, E. L.: Diagnostics of the fundus oculi, Troy, N. Y., 1920, Southworth Co.

7

which fit into the Contax camera body and consequently have gained about one-third more area in most of our views. Although narrow bands of light, sometimes brightly colored, have appeared at the very edge of many of our photographs magnified ×2½, we feel this is a small price to pay for the noticeably larger field of view, as in eyes in which the lesion still crowds the edge of the field.

We have found the ×5 magnification views of special value in recording fine details, such as, for instance, microaneurysms, vessel wall details, pigment distribution, and fine neovascularization. Photographic artifacts are fewer in these high-magnification pictures, partly because the edges of the total view are masked off by the rectangular frame within the film holder.

The true curvatures of the posterior coats of the eye do not show in our stereoscopic pictures. The total field is flattened because of the method used to gain the marked stereoscopic parallax. We do not consider this a detriment since all deviations from the normal curvature of the structures are represented by proportional deviations from the flat projection in the pictures.

Quantitative stereoscopic effect has not been achieved by our method, but the qualitative effect is marked, and it is dependable. If a feature appears elevated, it is certainly elevated in the eye; if it appears depressed (concave), the condition does exist in the eye. Only the easily identified error of mounting the stereoscopic views in reverse can give a false depth effect. Retinal vessels seen beyond the choroidal pattern, etc. are obvious clues to improper mounting. Therefore, there is little reason for doubting the validity of information presented in good stereophotographs.

The greater amount of information regarding the location of lesions in specific tissues or their localization within a tissue, such as opacities in the deep vitreous, nerve fiber layer, or deeper layers of the retina, is amazing by comparison with the simple maplike projection in two-dimensional pictures. Very little, if any, of the depth localization of lesions is sacrificed in the stereophotographs herein, even though the magnification is slightly reduced. The pictures still exemplify the kind of records which can be made. Furthermore, they should suggest the possibility that such records should be made of many patients who have diseases involving the fundus of the eye. Such pictures are hardly more difficult for an experienced photographer to make than single, two-dimensional pictures. Eventually, the practice of making stereophotographs could become widespread.

Such an accumulation of stereophotographs would have been impossible without the wholehearted cooperation of the entire staff of our Department. They have put their records and pictures at our disposal, and we wish to thank them for their contribution. Special thanks are due to Dr. Alson E. Braley, our chief, without whose enthusiastic support this book could never have been written. We are also indebted to many members of our hospital staff for letting us photograph their patients. We appreciate especially the cooperation of Dr. W. Kirkendall, who has put many of the photographs of his hypertensive patients at our disposal.

We owe special gratitude to the members of the Medical Illustration Department of the Veterans Administration Hospital in Iowa City. Under the direction of Mr. Charles Deutsch, they have helped us obtain the excellent photomicrographs. Their unceasing cooperation is greatly appreciated.

Finally, we wish to acknowledge the patience and understanding of Otty and Sally, who have borne with us during many hours of work while preparing the pictures and the manuscript.

Frederick C. Blodi
Lee Allen

Contents

Stereoscopic manual of
the ocular fundus
in local and systemic disease

Photographic method

The value of stereoscopic pictures of the fundus such as in this book should be self-evident. The same characteristics which make them superior to two-dimension pictures as records of cases also make them valuable in diagnosis. Frequently, they reveal important facts not seen during direct examination of patients. The effect of viewing the stereoscopic photographs is fundamentally like that of binocular indirect ophthalmoscopy, but with added advantages. High magnifications are easily achieved, and the photographs hold still for prolonged study of details. The broad, fully illuminated field in the photographs gives a more comprehensive view than can be appreciated at any one moment with a slit-lamp biomicroscope (although the latter remains indispensible for details which only an optical section can furnish).

The method by which the pronounced depth effect in these pictures is achieved has been described in detail in a paper entitled "Ocular fundus photography."[*] Another paper, "Steroscopic fundus photography with the new instant positive print films,"[†] describes the accessory to the fundus camera and the procedure by which it is possible to take pictures on Polaroid films for study at the time of examination of a patient.

Stereoscopic fundus photographs are only slightly more difficult to make than single, two-dimensional pictures if a systematic procedure is established and followed implicitly. Extra exposures to "play safe" in getting one good pair are not necessary except in rare cases which are easily

---

[*]Allen, L.: Ocular fundus photography, Am. J. Ophth. **57**:13-28, 1964.

[†]Allen, L.: Stereoscopic fundus photography with the new instant positive print films, Am. J. Ophth. **57**:539-543, 1964.

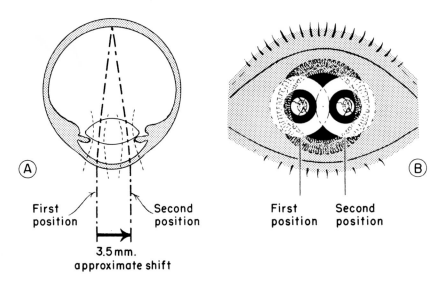

First position Second position

3.5 mm.
approximate shift

First position Second position

Diagram 1. Principles involved in the cornea-induced parallax method. **A,** Cross section of the eye showing the path of image and alignment of the camera for each of the two pictures required for stereopsis. **B,** Front view of the eye showing the position of the ring of light from the camera relative to the pupil for each of the two exposures. (**B** modified from Allen, Lee: Ocular fundus photography, Am. J. Ophth. **57:**13, 1964.)

recognized by the poor appearance of the images in the viewer of the camera.

We know of no fundus camera commercially available which can take both photographs of the stereoscopic pair simultaneously. Such a device would be most desirable because quantitative stereoscopy would automatically be possible, as has been achieved by Donaldson[*] with what must be a prototype of such a camera. Since this is not available to us, we must be content for the present to take the two pictures in close succession under conditions as well controlled as possible. It is, therefore, necessary to define clearly the basic principle by which a close consistency of the stereoscopic effect must be achieved.

Only the *cornea-induced parallax* method is used, the camera being directed through one side of the well-dilated pupil for the first exposure and then, without any angulation, moved to a parallel position on the other side of the pupil for the second exposure. This principle is shown in Diagram 1. Previous methods used slight rotation of the subject's eye or angulation of the camera or a combination of these. Such methods are difficult to systematize so that the amount of stereoscopic effect is erratic and usually minimal. A number of photographs published as stereoscopic views can be seen to have only a pseudostereoscopic effect based solely upon the appearance in depth of a reflection of the camera's light source, out in front of the retina. Such haphazard methods should be discarded in favor of the more controllable cornea-induced parallax method.

The original transparencies from which the copies included in this book

---

[*]Donaldson, D. D.: The eye in systemic disease, Scientific Exhibit, Meeting of the American Academy of Ophthalmology and Otolaryngology, Oct. 20-25, 1963.

were made were taken at either of two fixed magnifications, $2\frac{1}{2}\times$ (circular outline) and $5\times$ (rectangular outline) with the modern Zeiss fundus camera. It seems reasonable to believe that comparable pictures could be taken with other fundus cameras, especially if their illuminating systems can supply enough well-controlled light to the fundus when the camera is directed through the periphery of the dilated pupil. We highly recommend that those who have other types of cameras try the cornea-induced parallax method so that they, too, can take advantage of fine stereoscopic records.

Photographic imperfections and striking artifacts

The original photographs were taken on the effectively grainless Kodachrome II, daylight type, A.S.A. speed 25/3°, 35 mm. transparency film. It has several fine qualities, and we recommend it for fundus photography. However, its speed, wide latitude, fine resolution of detail, and color sensitivity, especially in the blue range, are such that photographic artifacts relating to the illumination, position and alignment of the camera and of the subject's eye can appear more frequently than when other types of film are used. We have therefore, found it necessary to modify the Zeiss camera slightly to reduce the chances of artifacts and to minify their importance when they cannot be avoided. The modifications will be de-described after a brief review of the nature of the most common photographic artifacts and faults in technique.

Improper focus

Poor resolution of the image upon the film obviously can be the result of imperfections in the optical media of the subject's eye. This cause is easily recognized and accepted as uncorrectable if all adjustments of the camera have been made correctly and yet the image in the sidearm focusing viewer cannot be sharply resolved at any position of the film-focusing knob. Single frame pictures of such indistinct subjects are usually very disappointing, whereas stereoscopic pictures in the same cases frequently record and reveal worthwhile information.

By contrast, if the image in the sidearm viewer is sharp and with good color and value contrasts but the image on the finished picture is less sharply focused, the fault can be corrected. Such imperfect results are more common with young photographers with very active ocular accommodations than with older photographers and are usually due to improper presetting of the focusing lens in the sidearm viewer. Even though such young persons follow the instructions for adjusting the focusing lens given in the manual furnished with the camera, they can still set the focus at the wrong level. If poorly focused pictures continue to occur after careful attempts to reset the focusing viewer, the determination of the truly correct setting can be made by paralyzing the photographer's accommodation with a cycloplegic drug. Then the viewing lens should be focused upon the cross hairs and the scale reading recorded for subsequent reference. If the photographer intends to wear spectacles during photography, he must wear them while making the determination—and obviously he must always wear them for the photography, unless another determination is made without them.

The photographer must perfect his ability to judge when the cross hairs in the viewer are in sharpest focus at the same time as the particular feature of interest in the image of the fundus.

Astigmatism can cause the image to be in focus along one meridian and blurred along the opposite. If the camera does not have corrective crossed cylinders for canceling this defect, as does the modern Zeiss, fairly satisfactory pictures can be made through the subject's spectacles or a cylindrical trial lens. Reflections from such accessory lenses must be avoided by slight tilting of the frames.

Aberrations caused by irregularities in curvature of the subject's crystalline lens or cornea usually cannot be corrected. The images from some highly myopic eyes are likely to be in focus only in the center of the view while objects toward the edge can appear radially elongated. These effects can be magnified if the camera is at other than an optimum distance from the eye. They can be reduced to a minimum by searching for the best possible distance.

One edge of image shadowed

Rarely, unequal illumination across the image can be caused by optical irregularities in the subject's eye, and it may or may not be possible to correct this by careful alignment of the camera.

Most commonly, shadowing of one edge of the image is due to the iris blocking off part of the illumination. Such uneven lighting is disturbing in single two-dimensional pictures, but it is remarkable how little it is noticed if it appears in one picture of a stereoscopic pair. This is fortunate because one shadowed edge in one picture may be unavoidable if the subject's pupil is irregular or does not dilate well and if an attempt is still made to achieve good stereoscopic effect in spite of the problem.

The shadow can be made worse by having the camera too close or too far from the subject's eye. If the presence of a shadow is recognized during focusing, an attempt should be made to find the optimum distance and thereby reduce the shadow as much as possible.

The shadowing will not be dark enough or extensive enough to be noticeable in most eyes in which the optics are nearly symmetrical and when an 8 mm. pupil is possible. When a shadow is seen encroaching upon the view, the camera can be moved to a point not so far from the center of the pupil. Furthermore, about the time the shadow of the iris begins to be noticeable during the shift to achieve the cornea-induced parallax, a point is reached where it is no longer possible to keep good resolution of detail in the image even with readjustment of the image-focusing knob. Therefore, it becomes doubly desirable to shift alignment very slightly toward the optically better area nearer the center of the pupil.

Bright ring-shaped or meniscus-shaped reflection from cornea

The most obvious artifact of illumination is a bright, warm, white reflection of the light source in the camera from the surface of the

16

cornea. In the modern Zeiss camera, it usually is meniscus-shaped and can be found at any meridian around the periphery of the view. In some subjects it can appear as a complete white ring encircling the view because it is a catoptric image of a ring-shaped aperture in the illuminating system.

If the entire ring is seen, it is eliminated by moving the camera farther away from the subject's eye. Slowly the ring expands and moves off the edges of the view. From the instant the ring is no longer seen, the camera usually should be moved still a bit farther from the eye to ensure that a portion of the ring will not reappear unexpectedly at the moment the photographic exposure is made.

The meniscus form of this catoptric image appears when the camera is both too close to the eye and slightly decentered from the optical axis of the subject's eye. If the camera is decentered to the photographer's left, the meniscus will appear on the left side of the picture; if decentered to the right, on the right side; if decentered upward, it will appear at the top, etc. If our interest here were in regard to single two-dimensional pictures, we would instruct that the reflection be eliminated by centering the axis of the camera and eye and moving the camera away slightly. But, for stereoscopic views the meniscus must be dealt with differently, because the camera is intentionally decentered. Here, we may keep the meniscus in the view and eliminate it by moving the camera away from the subject. As this is done, the reflection broadens, loses its sharp edges, and gradually decreases in intensity until it disappears or, at least, cannot be distinguished in the camera viewer. The sensitive color film might still pick up a faint haze at this point, but further movement of the camera toward the edge of the pupil, required by the stereoscopic technique, will truly eliminate it.

The illuminating system in the Zeiss fundus camera has been designed to avoid reflections from the central cornea and anterior lens substance. However, the light must "fan" out, once the level of the pupil is passed, in order to cover the retina with an even distribution of light. Therefore, some of the posterior crystalline lens substance and posterior capsule, as well as the vitreous body, is being flooded with light in the path of the image of the fundus as it emerges toward the camera. If there are even fine lens opacities, as in patients with diabetic cataract, irregularities in the capsule, or vitreous opacities, light will be dispersed by these features toward the camera, along with the image of the retina. This kind of "fogging" becomes worse if the camera is placed too far from the subject's eye. Therefore, if it appears, the camera should be moved toward the subject to reduce or eliminate it.

Luminous orange-colored area in image

Prismatic color separations due to the bending of light by the cornea and crystalline lens can show at the very edge of the pictures without being objectionable. However, there are positions of the camera in which the illuminating beam is affected prismatically so as to throw spots of luminous orange "glow" farther into the picture area. This color moves across the image opposite to the lateral and vertical movements of the camera and is easily and quickly eliminated from view by minor movements of the camera in almost any direction—laterally, vertically, or axially.

•   •   •

The most troublesome of all the photographic artifacts just described are the bright ring or meniscus-shaped catoptric image and the gray-blue haze which occur at opposite ends of the movement of the camera toward or away from the subject's eye. Between these extremes is an area of "leeway" within which neither defect appears—at least in certain apparently normal subject's eyes. The area is very narrow at best, and, unfortunately, it is even narrower in many abnormal eyes. In a few eyes there is no free area between the artifacts, and one or the other must be accepted in the picture. This is as true for single two-dimensional pictures as for stereoscopic views. This feature of the Zeiss camera has become especially troublesome since the introduction of the highly sensitive Kodachrome II film. We do not know if this is true of any instrument beside the modern Zeiss camera, but it would seem logical that there are similar problems with others due to basic problems of camera design.

It is possible to modify the Zeiss camera slightly in order to increase the free area and, therefore, the "leeway" for minor misalignments of the camera. These modifications are not only desirable in order to get good pictures in some eyes, where such would not otherwise be possible, but also to save a great deal of the photographer's time in adjustments to avoid the photographic artifacts. We have made five modifications which have reduced our problems so much that we highly recommend them to others. We further recommend that these be made by Carl Zeiss, Inc. or by a skilled instrument maker.

Camera modifications

1. Place an accessory mask in the illuminating system as shown in Diagram 2 so that less of the posterior lens and vitreous substances will be illuminated in the path of the emerging fundus image. This will, in effect, reduce the chances of having either the meniscus-shaped or ring-shaped catoptric image or the blue-gray haze appear in the pictures.

Cut, with reasonable care, a black paper disk 6.0 mm. in diameter. Across the center of the disk, glue two pieces of #60 black sewing thread at right angles to each other. Cut each of the four arms of the thread to about 8.0 mm. in length. Place a small piece of adhesive tape across each arm of the thread, near the end (do not use cellophane tape). The mask is then ready to install as illustrated.

Remove the aperture knob and the side plate of the camera and turn the aperture diaphragm wheel until the #7 (14 mm. diameter) aperture is accessible from both sides. Hold the black paper disk (accessory mask) in the center of the aperture on the side away from the light source, stretch one of the threads across the opening, and fasten the ends with the adhesive tape against the surface of the diaphragm wheel. Stretch and fasten the other thread in the same way. Move the ends of the threads if necessary for reasonably accurate centering of the mask within the aperture.

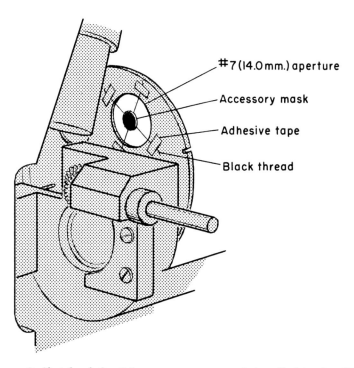

#7 (14.0 mm.) aperture

Accessory mask

Adhesive tape

Black thread

Diagram 2. Sketch of the 6.0 mm. accessory mask installed in the #7 aperture of the diaphragm wheel of the modern Zeiss fundus camera. (Adapted from Allen, Lee: Ocular fundus photography, Am. J. Ophth. **57**:13, 1964.)

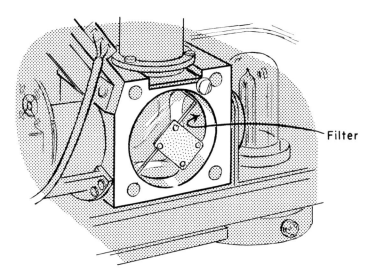

Filter

Diagram 3. Sketch locating the position for the installation of an 81a Wratten filter in the modern Zeiss fundus camera.

This installation may be relatively permanent, but it is hoped that the camera manufacturer will eventually make a still more permanent accessory available.

2. Install an 81a Wratten gelatin filter or, better yet, its glass equivalent in the electronic flash portion only of the illuminating system as shown in Diagram 3 to reduce the amount of blue component which is excessive for Kodachrome II film. The filter must not be placed so that it will reduce blue in the focusing light from the incandescent bulb, for this would make it even more difficult to recognize in the focusing viewer or anticipate the appearance of any blue-gray haze which might be recorded in the photograph. The filter may be placed anywhere between the underside of the inclined glass plate (which correlates the focusing and the photographic light paths) and the first condenser lens assembly closest to the electronic flash tube. It may be held in place with adhesive tape or other convenient means.

3. Install a special fixation device so that the patient may be presented with a fixation object projected optically to his far point of relaxation of accommodation. This must be done because the subject must have complete cycloplegia as well as dilatation of the pupil for consistently sharp focus of the photographic images. The subject cannot hold his eye steady if he is expected to look at a fixation object that is completely out of focus, which is true for the fixation light with which the camera is originally equipped.

If a special fixation device is not eventually made available by the camera manufacturer, the fixation device of the Haag-Streit "900" slit lamp may be adapted. A diagram of such an adaptation, with the critical dimensions, is shown in Diagram 4.

4. Move the camera housing backward 38.0 mm. on the supporting arm as described by Stenstrom,* using a one-fourth inch thick aluminum plate as an extension, as shown in Diagram 5. This modification places the focused ring of light, by which the camera is positioned relative to the cornea and pupil, upon the center of rotation of the camera's supporting arm. Thus, once the camera is correctly positioned, as directed in the manufacturer's instruction manual, the horizontal meridian of the subject's eye can be scanned for 90° without any appreciable movement of the joy stick. Equally important, there is room to shift the Haag-Streit "900" fixation target from one eye to the other without clumsy, distracting manipulations which would be necessary if the camera were in its original forward position.

• • •

The modifications alone do not guarantee the finest results. Artifacts of illumination can still appear occasionally in the photographs of abnormal eyes, even with the greatest of care in adjustment, but the chances of this are greatly decreased. Careless technique, on the other hand, can introduce artifacts in a large percentage of pictures.

---

*Stenstrom, W. J.: A modification of the new Zeiss fundus camera, Arch. Ophth. **64**:935, 1960.

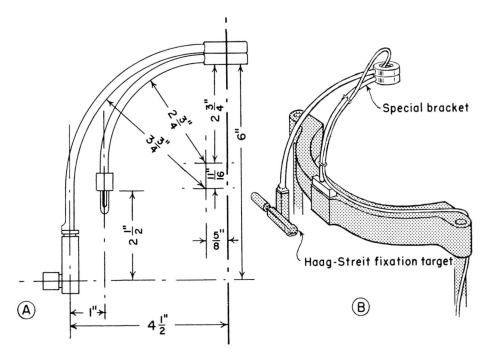

A

B

Special bracket

Haag-Streit fixation target

Diagram 4. Adaptation of the Haag-Streit "900" fixation device to the Zeiss camera. **A,** Mechanical drawing with essential dimensions for special bracket. **B,** Sketch of fixation device on special bracket in place on the forehead rest of the Zeiss fundus camera. (Adapted from Allen, Lee: Ocular fundus photography, Am. J. Ophth. **57**:13, 1964.)

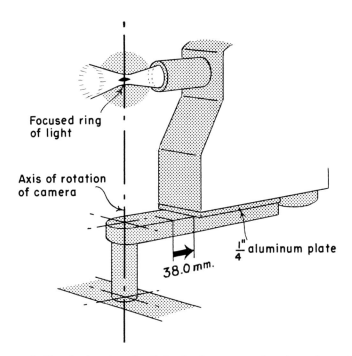

Focused ring of light

Axis of rotation of camera

$\frac{1}{4}''$ aluminum plate

38.0 mm.

Diagram 5. Sketch showing the Zeiss fundus camera housing relocated 38.0 mm. backward on the supporting arm to make the focused ring of light fall upon the axis of rotation for horizontal scanning. Aluminum plate required for the modification is indicated. (Adapted from Allen, Lee: Ocular fundus photography, Am. J. Ophth. **57:** 13, 1964.)

Photographic procedure

A well-conceived photographic procedure must be established and followed implicitly. This includes correct preparation of the patient as well as thoughtful handling of the camera. We have developed a systematic procedure which works very well for us and which we present here in detail. The number of steps listed may seem formidable and give the impression that they would be time consuming. Actually many of these are checks and doublechecks which take only one or two seconds each. A whole page of instructions (for instance, on manipulation of the camera) may take only four or five seconds actually to do. And by following the steps with understanding rather than using purely intuitive, haphazard approaches a great deal of time and film will be saved.

Preparation of the subject

The subject's eye must have complete cycloplegia in order to hold the image of the fundus at a fixed level during the focusing of the camera and the exposure of the film.

The pupil must be as wide as possible up to 8.0 mm. in diameter; otherwise, the stereoscopic effect will be limited.

The pupils of some diabetic patients and darkly pigmented subjects may be difficult to dilate well. Whatever drops are used, they may need to be repeated.

Cyclogyl, 1%, is a very satisfactory drug for producing both cycloplegia and dilatation. This may be reinforced with 1 drop of 10% Neo-Synephrine in viscous solution (Mono-drop) if necessary. If only shorter-acting drugs are preferred, the following are recommended, to be administered as noted:

1 drop of 1% Mydriacyl—*wait two or three minutes*
1 drop of 1% Mydriacyl—*followed immediately by*
1 drop of 10% Neo-Synephrine in **viscous** solution.

Photograph the eye after twenty-five or thirty minutes—not longer unless reinforcing drops must be used, in which case another ten or fifteen minutes may be required.

Other short-acting drugs have not proved satisfactory for photography even though they may have been considered excellent for direct ophthalmoscopic examination. Especially, Neo-Synephrine in aqueous solution *must never be used* because in many subjects it disturbs the corneal epithelium enough to reduce markedly the sharpness of the images in the pictures.

For those who may be unduly concerned about the possibility of causing an attack of angle-closure glaucoma by wide dilatation of the pupil, it must be pointed out that such danger is statistically insignificant. The exceptions are surveys in which groups of patients with known or suspected glaucoma are photographed. Tests for glaucoma may be made before and after photographing such patients. However, photographing must not immediately follow any test in which an instrument has been placed against the center of the surface of the cornea. Since the corneal epithelium will have been disturbed, several hours should elapse while the epithelium returns to normal. Otherwise the photographic image will not be sharply resolved.

The subject should be told of his role in the photography—that two closely related pictures must be taken and that he must remain exactly in one position until both exposures have been made.

The assistant

An experienced assistant must be available to hold the eyelids of some subjects well out of the photographic area. The lids can prevent some of the illumination from reaching the fundus, and, in some positions, they can reflect light irregularly to "fog" the image. Sometimes a deep pool of tears along the lower lid margin must be pulled away from the photographic area of the pupil. The assistant can also help check on the position and alignment of the camera and advise when a noticeable error must be corrected.

Step-by-step outline of stereoscopic procedure

All adjustments of the camera placement, the aperture settings and lens scale settings on the camera, as well as all intensity knob settings on the power supply case, must be checked before beginning to take photographs of each subject. Generally, all dials and switch knobs should be returned to the average, routine positions. However, if marked spherical or cylindrical optical corrections for the subject's vision are known in advance, the appropriate accessory lens may be rotated into place or the cross-cylinders may be preset.

It is advisable to have a mental checklist such as the following:

1. See that the sidearm focusing viewer is properly set for the photographer.

2. Be sure the #7 aperture is in place in the illuminating system. (Never use any aperture but the #7 for color photography, since other apertures introduce photographic artifacts, even in peripheral areas for which some, especially the oval ones, seem to have been designed.)

3. Check or preset the cross-cylinder knob on top of the camera.

4. Check or preset the accessory spherical lens knob on the upper right-hand side of the camera.

5. Place the camera in approximate position for photographing either the right or the left eye.

6. Place the fixation target on the appropriate side of the head rest.

7. If the picture is to be taken at 2½× magnification, see that the accessory magnifying lens is *not* on the camera. If it is to be taken at 5× magnification, see that the 2× accessory magnifying lens* *is* in place.

8. Check that the relay cable to the electronic flash unit is plugged into the Contax camera body.

9. Wind the film if necessary.

10. Going to the power supply unit, set the focusing light intensity knob on #2. (Never use less intensity for color photography. Resist as far as possible the temptation to make exceptions to this rule, because low intensity does not reveal the artifacts which might appear in the photographs.)

---

*Available from Carl Zeiss, Inc., New York, N. Y.

11. Set the electronic flash intensity knob at II when using Koda-chrome II and when the picture is being taken at $2\frac{1}{2}\times$ magnification. Set it at IV if it is being taken at $5\times$ magnification. Only after long experience should the photographer digress from this routine. More pictures will be spoiled by guessing at variations in exposure than by keeping a fixed routine.

We repeat that the preceding list of steps may give the impression that such a routine would be very time consuming. Actually, it takes about fifteen seconds, on the average, to run this set of checks and make adjustments. If the routine is not established, records of cases will sometimes be so poor as to be almost worthless or time and film will be wasted before errors in settings are noticed and corrected.

12. Seat the subject comfortably before the camera. Have him place his chin solidly down upon the chin rest, close his teeth, and place his forehead firmly against the forehead rest. Ask him to hold this position through the two exposures needed for the stereoscopic picture—until he is told he may move.

13. Place the fixation target before the eye not being photographed and adjust the focus of the target until the subject reports that it appears sharp. Align the target by estimation to bring the area of interest in the subject's eye into approximately the correct alignment with the camera.

14. Position the camera carefully before the subject's eye according to the instructions in the Zeiss manual while looking past the camera to focus the ring of light within the area of the pupil. Bring the joy stick into a vertical position, making any adjustments of the camera base and head rest positions necessary to make this possible while keeping the ring of light in place.

15. Grasp the joy stick gently with the left hand—never the right hand. Lock the stick with a light, sensitive touch so as not to wear the lock unduly and so the camera will not jump when it is unlocked.

16. Operate the vertical adjusting knob and the film-focusing knobs with the right hand, and eventually use the right hand to trip the camera shutter for the exposure.

17. View the fundus through the sidearm focusing viewer and focus the image. If the area of interest is not within view, look around the camera and move and tilt the fixation target appropriately to bring it into view.

18. When the object of the picture is properly centered, look around the camera again and recenter the ring of light on the pupil.

19. Back in the viewer again, eliminate any artifacts of illumination which might be present, recalling the analysis of these given earlier in the chapter.

After careful focusing of the image at this point, a single exposure may be made if desired for use as an ordinary 2" $\times$ 2" lantern slide.

20. Tilt the joy stick slowly to the left to align the camera through the left side (the photographer's left) of the pupil for the first exposure

of the stereoscopic pair. If the meniscus of the catoptic image appears, stop the sidewise tilting of the joy stick momentarily and pull the camera a very slight bit farther from the subject's eye. The moment the meniscus fades to nothing, continue the shift of the camera sidewise. Usually this will not be far before the image darkens noticeably. Sometimes a point is reached where the image loses its sharp resolution and adjustment of the film-focusing knob will not return the sharpness. If so, shift the camera very slightly back toward the center of the pupil.

21. When the point is found where the first picture might be taken, do not yet make the exposure. First, tilt the joy stick slowly to the right, beyond alignment with the center of the cornea and on to a point near the right side (the photographer's right) of the pupil. Find the desirable position for the second picture of the stereoscopic pair on this side. Do not make an exposure.

In effect, the movements made in steps 21 and 22 predetermine for the photographer the positions in which the two related pictures should be taken. With experience, he will remember the "feel" of the distance embraced by the scanning movement (usually about 3.5 mm)* and the end points between which it is bracketed.

22. Tilt the joy stick again to the left, find the position for the first exposure, check out the artifacts of illumination, vertically and horizontally, sharpen the focus, and make the exposure.

23. Remind the subject: "Don't move."

24. Shift the camera to the right with the joy stick, check all items noted in step 23, and make the exposure for the second picture of the stereoscopic pair.

In order to complete the systematic character of the procedure, it is advisable to take, always, the pictures of the right eye first and the left eye second. Thus, record keeping is simplified and the pictures are most easily identified after development, since they will always appear in the same order on the roll.

Photographing nasal and temporal peripheries

Pictures in the superior and inferior peripheries are taken in the same manner as those in central areas just described. However, they are frequently a little difficult to take because the pupil is effectively a horizontal oval. Pictures in the lateral peripheries are taken differently. When the subject's eye is rotated to the side for photography of the nasal or temporal areas of the fundus, the iris appears effectively as a vertical oval. There is not enough distance across the horizontal diameter to allow enough shift to achieve any worthwhile parallax between the two pictures. However, a worthwhile shift can be made vertically as shown in Diagram 6.

Align and focus through the center of the pupil.

---

*This figure, based upon actual measurements with a new device, corrects the erroneous estimate of 5.5 mm. of movement given in previous publications.

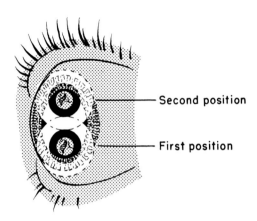

Diagram 6. Angular view of the eye in position for photographing the temporal periphery of the right eye or the nasal periphery of the left eye, showing the vertical shift between the position for the first and second exposures for stereoscopic pictures.

Shift downward and upward with the vertical adjustment knob to establish the end points effectively, as in steps 21 and 22.

If the picture is of the temporal side of the fundus of the right eye or the nasal side of the fundus of the left eye, take the first picture of the stereoscopic pair through the lower part of the pupil and the second through the upper part.

If the picture is of the nasal side of the fundus of the right eye or the temporal side of the fundus of the left eye, take the first picture through the upper part of the pupil and the second through the lower part.

Mounting the stereoscopic pictures

Use European-size mats* which have wider frames than the American.

Separate the pictures in such a way that the most distant feature, such as the cribiform plate in the nerve head, is separated exactly 63.0 mm. This makes for comfortable viewing and projection.

Adjust identical objects in the two pictures to the same height in the frames. Occasionally a subject will not have been able to prevent a noticeable vertical shift of the eyes between the two exposures. It is then necessary to clip the bottom of one film and sometimes the top of the other in order to adjust them for comfortable viewing. The final careful adjustment can be done by measurement from the lower edge of the aluminum mat, pushing the pictures upward or downward to corresponding levels.

The films may be fastened in place by bits of tape or by indenting with a needle point through the aluminum mat into the film in several places.

The views of the nasal and temporal peripheries must be rotated 90° in the mats because of the parallax having been achieved with a vertical rather than a horizontal shift of the camera.

Pictures of the temporal side of the fundus of the right eye and the nasal side of the fundus of the left eye must be rotated 90° to the right— the first picture taken being placed in the left-hand frame. Pictures of the

---

*Wide-frame aluminum stereoscopic mats; may be obtained from Karl Busch, 40 Schifferstrader St., Mannheim, Rheinau, West Germany.

nasal side of the fundus of the right eye and the temporal side of the fundus of the left eye must be rotated 90° to the left and, again, the first picture taken must be placed in the left-hand frame.

Since the rotation of these latter pictures places their narrow diameter horizontally, there is no need for using the wide-frame European mats. In fact, the narrower frame aluminum Stereo-Realist mats are ideal for these because, with them, the spracket holes along the sides of the film do not usually need to be covered with masking tape.

Viewing the stereoscopic pictures

Stereoscopic pictures of the fundus taken as described here are shown to best advantage in fine-quality hand stereoscopic viewers. The frames within these viewers may be filed out wider to reveal the full field of the European-size mat frames.

Good stereoscopic projectors with sufficient light and fine-quality aluminized screens, together with the best quality A. O. Polaroid spectacles, show the pictures surprisingly well to audiences of up to one hundred persons.

Normal fundus

Reel I-1. Adult fundus

The right eye of a 52-year-old white man. The patient came to our clinic for a routine refraction.

The photograph shows a normal optic nerve head. It is apparent that the mass of nerve fibers enters from the nasal side of the disc. The physiologic cup lies on the temporal side. On the temporal side is a pigment crescent lying at the margin of the papilla. Peripheral to this crescent is a small area of choroidal atrophy. The macula is normal. The vessels show changes consistent with the age of the patient, although the arteriovenous nicking seen in the lower area of the photograph is a sign of arteriolar sclerosis. In this crossing the arteriole, due to its thickened wall, seems to push the vein to one side, partly obscuring the blood stream in the underlying vessel.

Reel I-2. Fundus of child

The right eye of an 8-year-old white boy. In high magnification the disc can be seen to have a physiologic excavation on the temporal side. The mass of the nerve fibers enters on the nasal side of the disc. In the 8 o'clock meridian can be seen a cilioretinal artery which comes from the ciliary blood vessels and enters the retina around the edge of the papilla. This is a physiologic variation and may be of clinical importance. When the central retinal artery is occluded, this little arteriole running to the macula may still be patent. In the high magnification shown here, the nerve fibers themselves are hazily visible, especially on the nasal side of the disc.

28

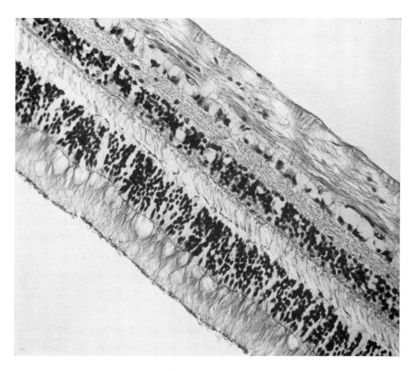

Figure 1. Histologic section through a normal retina. The three nuclear layers can be clearly distinguished. Toward the bottom of the photomicrograph are the rods and cones and their nuclei. Adherent to the rod and cone layer is the retinal pigment epithelium. This appears as a single layer of pigmented cells. In a normal eye this layer remains attached to the retina proper. Both layers shown here have been arti-factitiously detached from the choroid. The pigment content of the retinal pigment epithelium determines the color of the fundus. If the pigment content is excessive, the color of the fundus will be brownish or dark. If it is moderate, the fundus will have a uniform yellowish or orange color. If there is little or no pigment in this layer, the choroid will be visible.

Reel I-3. Fundus of young adult

The left eye of a 20-year-old white female student. The patient was referred to our clinic by the Department of Student Health to have her eyes examined as part of a routine physical examination.

The left optic nerve head is normal. On the temporal side of the disc is a crescent of choroidal atrophy. The retina itself shows a certain amount of shagreen often seen in young persons. The macula shows the reflex ring which outlines the area in which the retina is slightly thickened. In the center of this ring is the reflex of the foveal depression. Beneath it is a slight stippling of the pigment epithelium.

Reel I-4. Adult fundus

The left eye of a 45-year-old white man. The optic nerve head shows on its temporal margin a white crescent where choroid and pigment epithelium are absent and through which the sclera is visible. The macula is normal for the age of the patient, and the reflex so frequently seen in

29

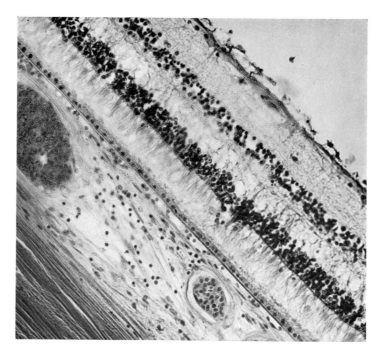

Figure 2. Cross section through an albinotic fundus. The retina is normal. There is no pigment in the retinal pigment epithelium, and the cells are, therefore, clearly discernible. Also there is no pigment in the choroid. In such a fundus the choroidal vessels can be seen clearly against the white background of the sclera.

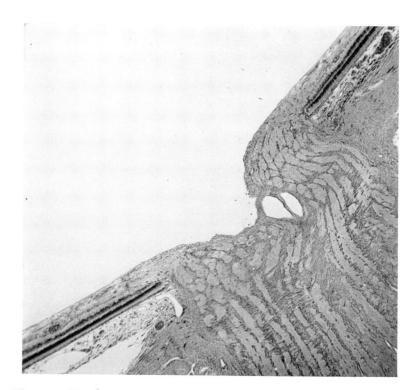

Figure 3. Histologic appearance of a normal optic nerve head. Its nasal side, which appears on the right side of this photomicrograph, is characterized by an accumulation of nerve fibers. On the temporal side (left side of the picture) fewer nerve fibers enter the optic nerve and the physiologic excavation extends toward that side.

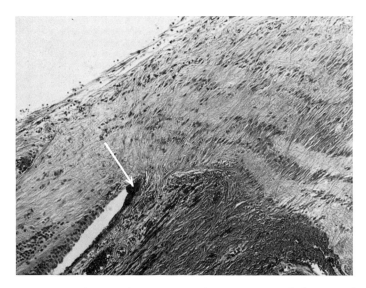

Figure 4. Accumulation of pigment in the pigment epithelium at the temporal border of the disc. This layer is thickened and deeply pigmented where it stops at the entrance of the optic nerve head.

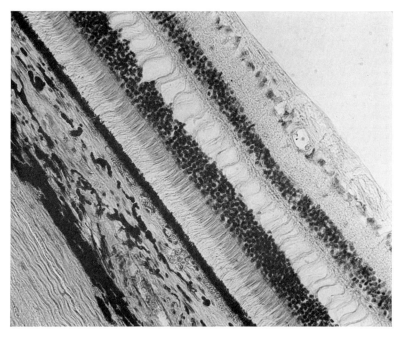

Figure 5. Cross section through a deeply pigmented fundus. The pigment epithelium can be seen as a jet black ribbon between the choroid and the retina. In the choroid itself there are also numerous pigmented cells which are more concentrated in the outer layer of this organ, invading the sclera.

young persons is no longer present. The vascular tree corresponds to the age of the patient.

Reel I-5. Adult fundus

The right eye of a 33-year-old white man. The patient came to our clinic because of a primary optic atrophy on the right side. The left eye was absolutely normal.

Here, the optic nerve head appears somewhat flat, and no definite physiologic excavation is present. The macula and the vascular tree correspond to the age of the patient.

Reel I-6. Adult fundus

The left eye of a 53-year-old white woman. The patient came to our clinic because of senile macular degeneration in the right eye. The left eye was completely normal.

The left optic nerve head itself is normal with a cilioretinal artery in the 3 o'clock meridian. The macula and the vascular tree correspond to the age of the patient.

Reel I-7. Fundus of Negro

The right eye of a 30-year-old Negro physician. Both eyes were completely normal.

The photograph shows a pigment sickle temporal to the disc. The whole fundus shows not only the dark background characteristic of a deeply pigmented person, but also the retinal shagreen peculiar to a young person.

Congenital
and
developmental diseases

Reel II-1. Medullated nerve fibers

The right eye of an 18-year-old Negro student. The patient was admitted to the Medical Clinic because of severe asthma. He had no complaints with his vision, and visual acuity was 6/6 in both eyes.

A routine examination of the fundi revealed this unusual mass of myelinated nerve fibers around the right optic nerve head. These medullated nerve fibers appear as grayish-white opacities lying in the most superficial layers of the retina. They characteristically end with a feathery border. They lie so close to the surface of the retina that they obscure even the large retinal vessels. In this instance they are so massive that they nearly encircle the entire circumference of the papilla, leaving only the temporal segment free. Usually they lie adjacent to the disc, but sometimes they can be found away from the disc. At the lower disc margin there is a clear interval between the disc and the opacities of the myelinated nerve fibers.

Such massive myelination resembles the fundus of some rodents (papilla leporina).

Reel II-2. Coloboma of choroid

The right eye of a 12-year-old girl. The patient was first seen in our clinic at the age of 5 years because of a left esotropia. This squint was apparently present since birth but had improved gradually. At 3 years of age the patient had suffered from encephalitis, and since then she has been mentally retarded. The coloboma of the right choroid had been noticed on her first visit.

When this photograph was taken, vision in the right eye was 6/21 and that in the left eye was 6/6. The left eye was absolutely normal.

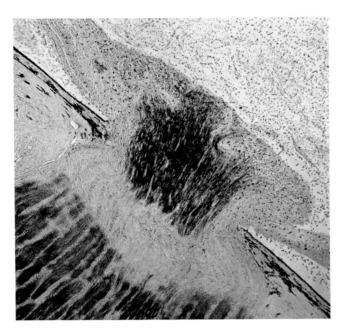

Figure 6. Myelinated nerve fibers in front of the cribriform plate. A myelin sheath stain was used, and in this photomicrograph the myelin appears as a black deposit. The myelinated fibers in the optic nerve are plainly visible. Then follows an interruption in the area of the cribriform plate. In front of it is another bundle of myelinated fibers.

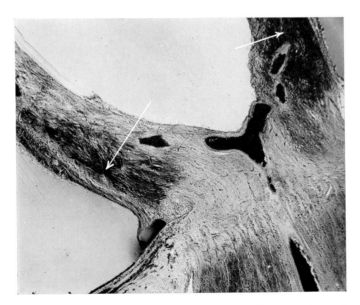

Figure 7. Another example of myelinated nerve fibers in the retina. Again, a myelin stain was used, and the myelinated fibers in the optic nerve can be seen in the right lower corner. Myelinated nerve fibers are visible on both sides in the detached retina.

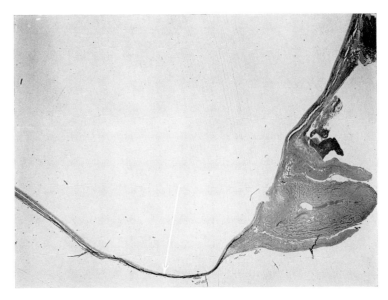

Figure 8. Low-power photomicrograph of a choroidal coloboma. The coloboma lies at the lower border of the figure, adjacent to the disc. In this area the coats of the eye are extremely thin and bulging outward. Peripheral to this area, choroid and retina appear again.

The right eye shows a huge excavated colobomatous area below the optic disc. Only the upper part of this coloboma is visible on the picture. In this area, retinal vessels can be seen dipping down, and no choroid is present. The retina seems to lie directly on the sclera. The coloboma does not reach the optic nerve, but the nerve itself is somewhat hazy in its outlines and has a horizontally oval shape. The coloboma itself was surrounded by a margin of pigmentation in the lower periphery.

Reel II-3. Coloboma of optic nerve

The right eye of a 4½-year-old white boy. At the age of 3 months, an iris coloboma was diagnosed in both eyes. When this child was 2 years old, he developed an esotropia of the right eye. Vision in the right eye was reduced to 6/30, and in the left eye it was 6/9.

The right fundus is pale and nearly albinotic. The disc is markedly elongated and enlarged. Most of the vessels to the retina come from the lower part of the disc, where they seem to emerge from a bottomless pit. Another branch of the central retinal vessels comes from the upper part of the elongated disc and also dips down deeply. The disc is surrounded by a margin of black pigment which is absent only in the lower segment. Around it is an area of choroidal atrophy.

Note: Light is reflected from the cornea into the right picture.

Reel II-4. Vessel loop into vitreous

The left eye of a 35-year-old white housewife. The patient was seen in the course of a population study for glaucoma. Both eyes were essentially

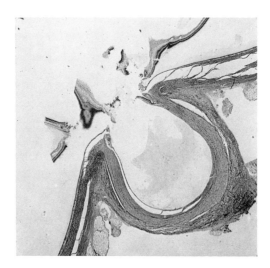

Figure 9. An unusually deep coloboma of the optic nerve head. The optic nerve itself was extremely atrophic.

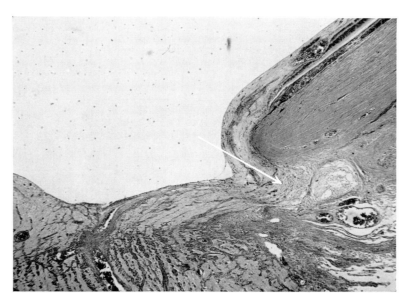

Figure 10. Histologic section through a mild coloboma of the optic nerve head or a so-called optic pit. On the right side of the photomicrograph the nerve fibers dip deep into the sclera at the margin of the papilla.

normal, and vision in both eyes was 6/6. She had never had any eye troubles in the past.

An incidental finding was this prominent vessel loop which extends from the left disc into the vitreous. The color of the vessel loop makes it a part of the venous system. The vessels go forward far into the vitreous, and they are twisted around each other. They have nothing to do with a persistent hyaloid artery which sometimes can be seen as a congenital anomaly as a stalk extending from the optic nerve head toward the posterior surface of the lens.

Reel II-5. Retinal fold

The left eye of a 65-year-old white woman. The patient was first seen at the age of 38 years, and at that time she stated that vision in the left eye had always been poor. Vision was 6/6 in the right eye and counting fingers at 3 feet in the left eye. The right eye was entirely normal, and the anterior segment of the left eye was normal.

The left fundus shows an extensive and high retinal fold extending from the disc toward the upper periphery. The nerve head itself cannot be seen, but the grayish-white mass which lies in the upper periphery is quite visible. This mass of connective and glial tissue is highly elevated and is still connected to the underlying retina. The retina at the base of this mass shows marked pigmentation. Similar areas of black hyperpigmentation alternating

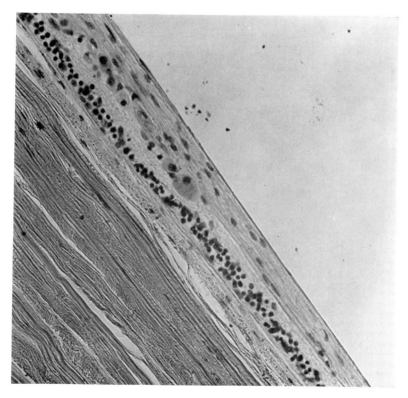

Figure 11. Histologic section through an eye with choroideremia. The retina is highly atrophic and thin. Neither pigment epithelium nor choroid is present.

with patches of depigmentation are also seen nasal to the fold and, in the lower part of the photograph, toward the optic nerve head.

Later in life this patient experienced an acute glaucomatous attack in both eyes for which she underwent a peripheral iridectomy. Later on, both lenses were extracted, and this picture was taken in the aphakic left eye. Vision in the left eye could not be improved. Vision in the right eye with aphakic correction remained 6/6.

Reel II-6. Choroideremia

The right eye of a 49-year-old white man. Since the age of 30 years, this patient had noticed a loss of central vision in both eyes. Even before that time he noticed that he had poor vision with reduced illumination. His maternal grandfather, as well as a male cousin on his mother's side, apparently had the same condition.

When this patient came to our clinic, vision in his right eye was reduced to 6/9 − 3 and that in the left eye to 6/12 + 3. The visual fields were markedly constricted. Even the 20 mm. target was seen at 1 meter within 5° of the fixation point. The electroretinogram was practically extinguished. The dark adaptation curve was markedly flattened, and after forty-five minutes the light sensitivity had increased by only 1 log unit. The fundus was nearly identical in both eyes.

This photograph shows a normal disc and nearly normal retinal vessels. There is an accumulation of pigment in the retina especially over the macula and also above and below it. Similar fine flakes of pigment can be seen nasally. In the central part of the picture the choroid is absent, and only the white reflex from the sclera can be obtained. There is, however, a pattern of choroidal vessels in the macular area and just temporal to the disc.

Reel II-7. Developmental macular degeneration

The right eye of a 30-year-old white woman. The patient had noticed distortion of vision one year previously. This was more marked in the left eye than in the right eye. The x-ray film of the skull was normal.

When the patient came to us, vision in the right eye was 6/6, and that in the left eye was 6/9–3. The anterior segments were normal. The left macular area showed some fine pigmentation.

The right macular area shows pronounced pigmentation deep in the retina. There are also some small areas of depigmentation present. The vascular tree is perfectly normal, and the optic nerve head is also normal.

The Amsler grid showed marked distortion in both eyes. The electroretinogram was normal. The patient stated that other members in her family also suffered painless progressive loss of vision fairly early in life.

Senile and
degenerative changes

Reel III-1. Beginning senile macular degeneration

The right eye of a 56-year-old woman. The patient came to our clinic for a presbyopic refraction. Vision in both eyes with correction was 6/6.

The photograph of the right fundus shows a normal disc with a choroidal atrophy as a temporal crescent. The vascular changes are consistent with the age of the patient. The arterioles show increased light reflexes, and there are some arteriovenous crossing phenomena where the thickened artery partially obscures the underlying vein. In the lower periphery of the photograph is the somewhat rare occurrence of an arteriole lying beneath the crossing vein.

The macula shows definite pathologic changes with a small area of depigmentation and a few patches of hyperpigmentation. Such a beginning senile macular degeneration may be compatible with good central vision.

Reel III-2. Senile macular degeneration

The right eye of a 62-year-old white man. The patient noticed slight deterioration of vision in both eyes for the last three years. The vision had been 6/9 in both eyes one year before this picture was taken. At present, vision in the right eye is reduced to counting fingers at 2 feet, and this cannot be improved. Vision in the left eye remains at 6/9. The patient is otherwise essentially healthy.

The macula of the right eye shows an area of hyperpigmentation in the center. This is surrounded by a wreath of small drusen. These drusen extend toward the periphery, but decrease there in number. The retinal

39

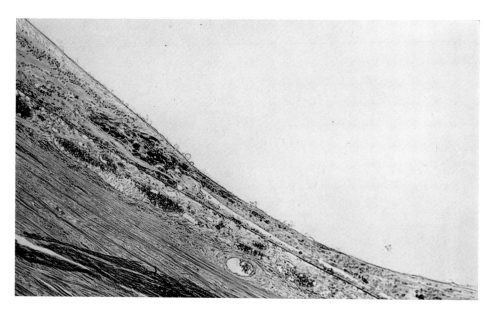

Figure 12. Senile macular degeneration. In the macular area there is marked atrophy of all the retinal layers. Here, the retina is replaced by a mass of pigmented glial tissue. The choroid beneath it is normal except for some thickening of its vessel walls.

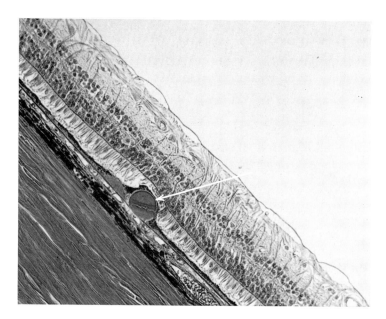

Figure 13. Histologic section through a senile druse. An accumulation of amorphous eosinophilic material can be seen on Bruch's membrane at the center of the picture. This is covered by pigment epithelium. The retina above it shows some atrophy of the rods and cones and a slight bowing of the external limiting membrane.

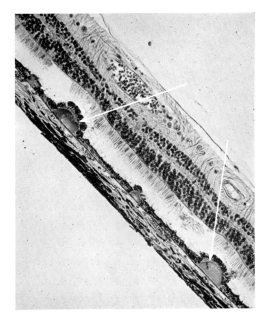

Figure 14. Another histologic section showing senile drusen. There are two such examples illustrated. On one of them, a hyperpigmentation of the retinal pigment epithelium can be noticed.

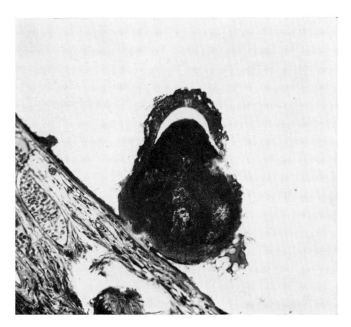

Figure 15. Another type of druse usually found in eyes with severe degenerative changes. In this instance the proliferation from Bruch's membrane is more uneven and partly calcified. In contrast to the so-called senile drusen, this is an example of a pathologic druse.

41

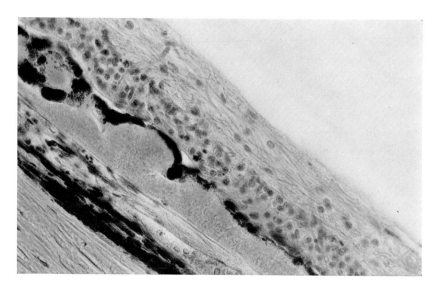

Figure 16. More diffuse proliferation of cuticular material from the pigment epithelium. This corresponds to the senile drusen, but it is more extensive and massive.

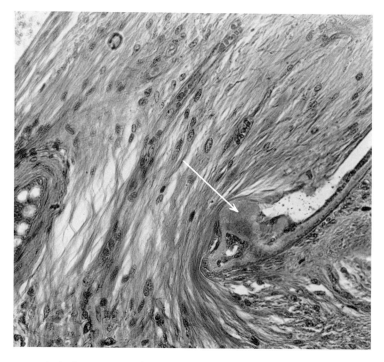

Figure 17. A druse situated near the end of Bruch's membrane at the margin of the optic nerve head. Here, again, an excrescence of hyaline material can be seen jutting forward from the pigment epithelium and impinging upon the nerve fibers as they enter the optic nerve.

arterioles show increased light reflexes, and there is an arteriovenous crossing phenomenon present above the disc.

Note: The stereoscopic effect in this picture is less than in most because minimal parallax resulted from inability to dilate the subject's pupil as widely as usual.

Reel III-3. Senile macular degeneration with drusen

The right eye of a 33-year-old white housewife. The patient came to our clinic because of a slight deterioration of vision in the left eye.

On admission, vision in the right eye was 6/6, and that in the left eye was 6/6 − 2. The pathologic findings were confined to the fundi.

This photograph shows the area just above the right macula. In the deeper parts of the retina are numerous punched-out, white-to-yellowish, atrophic areas. Some of these coalesce, and many of them are surrounded by a margin of hyperpigmentation. This is the characteristic opthalmoscopic picture of the so-called drusen or excrescences of Bruch's membrane. These lie deep to the retina and should not be confused with deep, waxy exudates. They are usually senile degenerative changes and cause visual disturbance only when they lie in the foveal area.

Reel III-4. Senile macular degeneration with crystals

The left eye of a 67-year-old white woman. The patient was referred to our clinic because of poor vision in both eyes. The eye findings were confined to the fundi. Vision in the right eye was reduced to 6/30 and that in the left eye to 6/21.

The blood cholesterol level was found to be 396 mg%. Because of this, the patient was put on a low cholesterol diet, but one year later the vision had not changed.

This is a photograph of the left macular area. In the center of it is an accumulation of crystals which lie in the retina itself. This mass of crystals is surrounded by a number of smaller areas of the same appearance. In addition, there are numerous drusen in the right lower corner of the picture.

Note: Corneal reflex is present in the upper edge of the left picture.

Reel III-5. Moderate myopia

The right eye of a 39-year-old white college professor. The patient came to our clinic for a check of his glasses. In both eyes he had a myopia of 8 diopters. With appropriate correction, the vision could be improved to 6/6 + 3 in both eyes. The positive eye findings were confined to the fundi.

The right eye shows a nearly albinotic fundus in which there is little pigment in either the pigment epithelium or the choroid. Consequently, the choroidal vascular pattern is easily visible. The disc is somewhat oblique and has a marked temporal crescent. There is also a cilioretinal artery in the 11 o'clock meridian at the disc. On the nasal side of the disc the retina is pulled over onto the papilla (supertraction).

Note: The light flare in the upper left-hand corner of the photograph **43**

is prismatic separation of the illumination due to improper alignment of the eye and camera.

Reel III-6. High myopia

The right eye of a 66-year-old white woman. The patient had had poor vision in the right eye for twelve years but began to notice some decrease in vision in the left eye. She had a myopia of about 13 diopters in each eye. Vision in the right eye could not be improved beyond counting fingers at 3 feet. In the left eye the vision could be improved to 6/21. The left fundus showed an extensive choroidal atrophy around the disc.

This is a photograph of the posterior pole of the right eye. The optic disc is oval, and it is surrounded by a large area of choroidal atrophy which extends primarily toward the temporal side. The entire fundus is blond. There is some retinal pigmentation below the disc. On the temporal side in the macula is another area of atrophy which appears white. These areas of choroidal atrophy occur frequently at the posterior pole of eyes with severe myopia. In addition, the macula contains an accumulation of black pigment. This is the so-called Fuchs' spot, which occasionally appears in the macula of patients with severe myopia, extinguishing central vision.

Note: This picture has distortion of the image at the edges related to the myopia. It must be assumed, however, that the irregularities in the

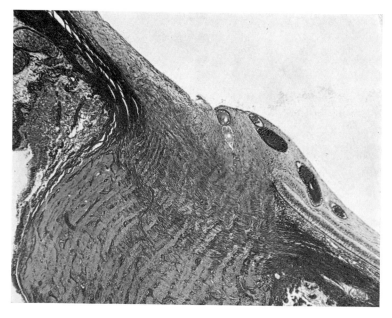

Figure 18. Cross section of an optic nerve head in severe myopia. The temporal margin (on the left side of the photomicrograph) is flat and the physiologic excavation is shallow. On that side, choroid, pigment epithelium, and retina do not reach the disc margin (temporal crescent). On the nasal side (the right side of the picture) the retina is pulled over onto the disc (supertraction). Remarkable is the short distance between the surface of the disc and the cribriform plate, making even a glaucomatous excavation appear rather shallow. This is one of the reasons why glaucoma is difficult to diagnose in eyes with severe myopia.

44

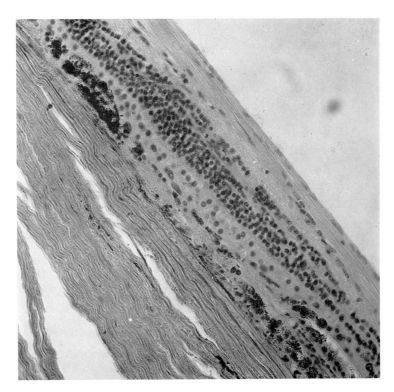

Figure 19. An area of severe chorioretinal atrophy due to high myopia. The choroid is nearly absent, and in the center the retinal pigment epithelium is also lacking. The retina is atrophic over that area. This would correspond to the white area seen with the ophthalmoscope as the transparent retina lies directly on the white-appearing sclera. This area is surrounded with a certain amount of hyperpigmentation of the pigment epithelium.

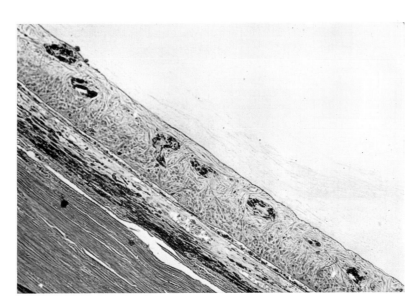

Figure 20. A typical case of retinitis pigmentosa. The retina is thin, and the layer of the rods and cones is absent. There is pigmentation in the retina which tends to accumulate around the blood vessels. The pigment epithelium is interrupted. The choroid is normal. There are no chorioretinal adhesions, and this distinguishes this type of degenerative disease or abiotrophy from a diffuse chorioretinitis.

45

plane of the sclera and choroid are real since retinal vessels can be seen to bridge smoothly across recessed areas.

Reel III-7. Retinitis pigmentosa

The left eye of a 39-year-old white engineer. The patient had no visual difficulties until seven years previously, when he noticed a gradual loss of peripheral vision. The central vision remained normal until about six months before he came to our clinic.

In addition, the patient developed some neurologic deficits, such as weakness of gait, numbness of the face, and loss of memory. He was seen by the Department of Neurology, and they suspected a beginning demyelinating disease.

When he came to us, vision in the right eye was 6/6, and in the left eye it could be improved to 6/21. The visual field of the right eye was definitely constricted, especially with small targets. In the left eye even large targets could not be seen outside of 10° from the fixation point.

The right eye was essentially normal with the exception of the fundus, which showed some abnormal pigmentation in the periphery. The left eye showed a posterior subcapsular cataract and a definite pallor of the disc. The retinal arterioles were attenuated, and there was massive retinal pigmentation. The retinal pigmentation was similar to that in the right eye but was more extensive.

The electroretinogram was extinguished on the left and subnormal on the right side. The dark adaptation curve did not show any scotopic response.

The photograph shows a peripheral area in the left eye. The most conspicuous feature is the accumulation of pigment in the superficial retina. This pigmentation tends to follow the outlines of small vessels and, therefore, occasionally assumes bone-corpuscle shape.

Optic nerve head

Reel IV-1. Primary optic atrophy

The right eye of a 4-year-old boy. When this child was 2 months old, he suffered numerous seizures and finally severe convulsions. When he was 3 months old, a craniotomy was performed after pneumoencephalography revealed a subdural collection of air. Subdural taps gave some xanthochromic fluid. During the operation, a subdural membrane was removed and some fluid drained. After the operation the patient developed fairly well, although there was some evidence of mental retardation.

Subsequent to the operation, the patient developed an esotropia of the right eye. Vision in the right eye was reduced to 1/60, while vision in the left eye was 6/15. The left eye was completely normal, although there was some questionable pallor of the optic nerve head.

The photograph shows the right optic nerve head which is sharply outlined but extremely pale. There is a conspicuous lack of small vessels and capillaries on and around the disc. The large retinal vessels appear normal, but the optic nerve head is flattened and the normal papilla (that is, the normal elevation of the nerve fibers in the area of the disc) is absent. The disc is surrounded by an area of hyperpigmentation on the upper and temporal side. Peripheral to that is a wide ring of choroidal atrophy in which the pigment epithelium is also absent. This ring appears, therefore, white.

Reel IV-2. Glaucomatous optic atrophy

The left eye of a 55-year-old man. The patient noticed blurring of vision in both eyes for the previous three to four months. He also saw colored haloes around white lights for about a year. He has had no pains in his eyes. The eyes were never red, nor was there any discharge. Occa-

47

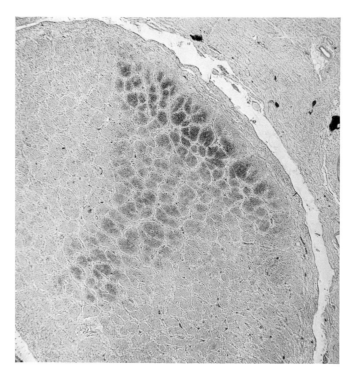

Figure 21. Cross section through an atrophic optic nerve. This is a myelin stain, and only a wedge-shaped sector of the optic nerve still shows myelin around the nerve fibers. The remaining nerve fibers are demyelinated and atrophic. The optic nerve itself is smaller than normal, and its sheaths are thickened.

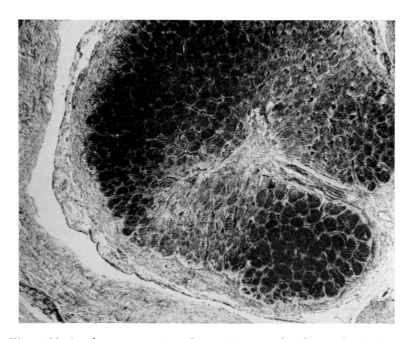

Figure 22. Another cross section of an optic nerve, but here a beginning atrophy is illustrated. The myelin stain shows that the large majority of fiber bundles still contain myelin, which appears black on this photomicrograph. Only in the central part of the optic nerve are some bundles demyelinated.

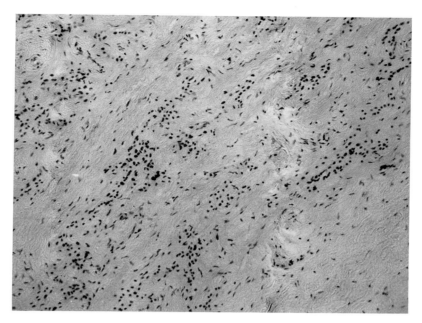

Figure 23. Transverse section through an atrophic optic nerve. The nerve fibers are replaced by an irregular proliferation of glial elements. There is also an increase in thickness of the connective tissue septa.

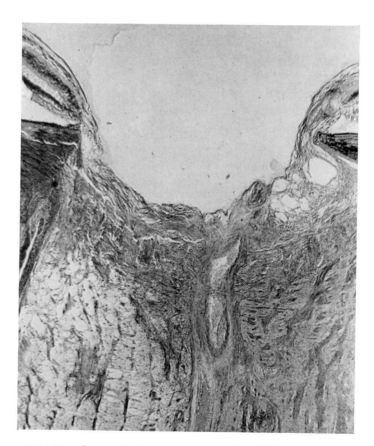

Figure 24. Far-advanced glaucomatous atrophy of the optic nerve. The glaucomatous excavation is complete, and there are hardly any nerve fibers left in front of the cribriform plate. The plate itself is bowed backward. The optic nerve back of the cribriform plate shows the cavernous type of optic atrophy on the left side of the photomicrograph. This atrophy occurs only in eyes with advanced glaucoma and is a type of mucoid degeneration of the optic nerve.

49

sionally the patient suffers from bitemperal headaches. It is interesting to note that his father is blind in both eyes because of glaucoma.

When the patient was seen in our clinic, vision in both eyes with correction was 6/9. The anterior segments were normal. Both optic discs showed rather deep excavations. The excavation in the left disc reaches the margin of the optic nerve head temporally and below. The nicking of the retinal vessels over the margin is plainly visible. The fundus itself has a tigroid appearance.

The intraocular pressure in both eyes varied between 25 and 30 mm. Hg. The visual fields showed nerve fiber bundle defects characteristic for glaucoma.

Reel IV-3. Glaucomatous optic atrophy

The left eye of a 14-year-old white boy. At an earlier age, the patient was aware of very poor vision in the left eye. Also, the left eye always appeared larger than the right eye. Occasionally he had some pain in the left eye.

When he came to our clinic, the right eye was entirely normal and vision was better than 6/6. The left eye was larger than the right eye and seemed to be bulging forward. Vision in that eye was reduced to light perception. The cornea was clear and the anterior chamber unusually deep. The intraocular pressure on the left side was 55 mm. Hg.

The optic nerve head on the left side shows a deep, nearly total excavation. The retinal vessels can be seen coming out from this deep cup, bending over the ridge of the excavation lying on the nasal side. Only a small rim of normal disc tissue remains.

Reel IV-4. Papilledema with meningitis

The left eye of a 24-year-old white student. The patient had become seriously ill five years before we saw him. He experienced severe headache, fever, stiff neck, and tender muscles. At that time the cerebrospinal fluid showed numerous white blood cells and an increased protein content. He was first treated for poliomyelitis and later on for suspected viral encephalitis. Six months later coccidioidomycosis was diagnosed for the first time. The organism could be cultured from the cerebrospinal fluid on several occasions. The patient had repeated attacks of nausea, vomiting, lethargy, and weakness. He received numerous courses of amphotericin B. When this photograph was taken, the pressure in the cerebrospinal fluid was still increased. The fluid was slightly opaque, and the cell count was 285, with a total protein of 370 mg%. The blood coccidioides titer was 4+.

When the patient was seen in our clinic, vision in both eyes was 6/9, and the pathologic changes were confined to the eyegrounds. Visual fields showed constriction for small targets and definitely enlarged blind spots.

The photograph of the left disc shows a markedly elevated papilla. The elevation measures about 3 diopters. The outlines of the disc are hazy and indistinguishable. The vessels on and around the disc are markedly dilated. A few superficial hemorrhages are present, especially at 12 o'clock.

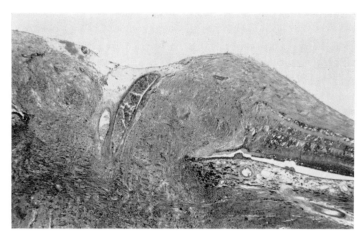

Figure 25. Cross section through an optic nerve with pronounced papilledema. The optic nerve fibers in front of the cribriform plate are swollen and bulging forward. The physiologic cup has disappeared. There is dilatation of the vessels, and the retina has been pushed aside by the swollen nerve fibers. Normally, the retinal elements reach the margin of the optic nerve in line with Bruch's membrane and the choroid. In cases of papilledema the retinal elements are pushed laterally, as is illustrated in this case. In addition, there is a slight peripapillary retinal detachment recognizable by the accumulation of some stainable fluid between the retina and pigment epithelium. This circumscribed detachment contributes to the clinical finding of an enlarged blind spot. In addition, there is an enlargement of the subarachnoid space of the optic nerve behind the sclera. This frequently occurs when the papilledema is due to increased intracranial pressure.

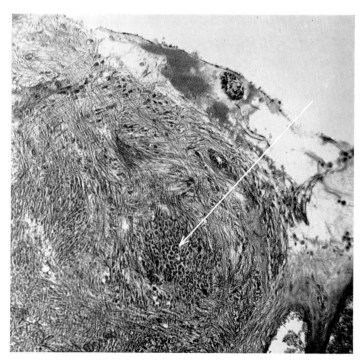

Figure 26. High-power field of Figure 25. On the left side an accumulation of cytoid bodies can be seen in the optic nerve head close to its surface. These cytoid bodies are similar to those occurring in the nerve fiber layer of the retina and are probably due to anemic infarcts in that area. They are more fully discussed and illustrated in Figures 47 and 48.

Reel IV-5. Papilledema with glioma

The right eye of a 6-year-old white girl. On a school examination, the patient was noted to have decreased visual acuity in the right eye. At the same time, her mother noted that the right eye was somewhat more prominent than the left eye. She had no pain or any other symptoms.

When the child came to our clinic, vision in the right eye was reduced to 6/60. The left eye was entirely normal. With the exophthalmometer the right eye had a reading of 20 and the left eye a reading of 12. An x-ray film of the orbit showed that the right optic foramen was slightly larger than the left one.

The photograph of the right optic nerve head shows a marked elevation of the papilla. This elevation measures about 3 to 4 diopters. The veins are somewhat enlarged, but there are no hemorrhages or exudates present on the nerve head.

The visual field on the right side shows a large central scotoma. The visual field on the left side was normal.

A Krönlein exploratory approach to the right orbit was done, and a markedly thickened and hardened optic nerve was found and excised. Histologic examination revealed this to be a glioma of the optic nerve. Since this tumor extended into the optic foramen, one week after the first operation the rest of the optic nerve up to the chiasm was resected by a frontal craniotomy. The patient recovered without any difficulties.

Reel IV-6. Papilledema with pseudotumor cerebri

The left eye of a 30-year-old white housewife. The patient came first to the hospital because of severe headache and visual disturbances. She was slightly obese but otherwise appeared healthy. When she came to our clinic, vision in both eyes was better than 6/6. The positive eye findings were confined to the optic nerve heads.

The photograph of the left fundus shows the optic nerve head elevated about 3 to 4 diopters. The papilla is somewhat yellowish in color. No hemorrhages or venous congestion was noted at this time, although both had been present previously.

The visual fields were normal with the exception of an enlargement of the blind spots. The patient was admitted to the Neurology Department. No neurologic deficit was found. An x-ray film of the skull was normal. The cerebrospinal fluid had a definitely enlarged pressure with increased protein content but normal cell count.

The patient was put on a diuretic, and the symptoms improved. She was followed for over five years, during which time the eye findings did not change materially.

Reel IV-7. Pseudopapilledema

The left eye of a 25-year-old medical student. The patient was completely normal and had no difficulties of any kind. This unusual eye finding was discovered in his junior year when one of his fellow students looked

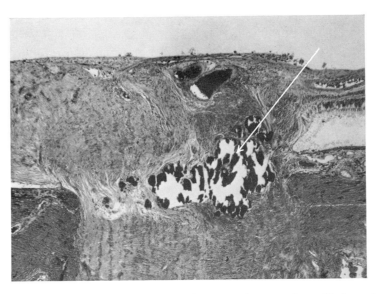

Figure 27. One of the pathologic substrates of a pseudopapilledema is an accumulation of hyalinized or calcified material in the optic nerve head. These are the so-called drusen of the optic nerve head. Their origin is not well understood. They may develop from accumulations of glial elements as they occur in the gliotic plaques of tuberous sclerosis. On the other hand, they are sometimes present as congenital anomalies without any associated systemic defects. If they lie superficially in the nerve substance, they are visible with the ophthalmoscope, and such a case is illustrated on Reel VII-7. If they lie deep in the substance, they cannot be seen and only their effect (namely, a pseudopapilledema) can be appreciated. In this instance the calcified nodule lies close to the cribriform plate. A great deal of the calcium has dropped out during the preparation of the slide, leaving an empty space.

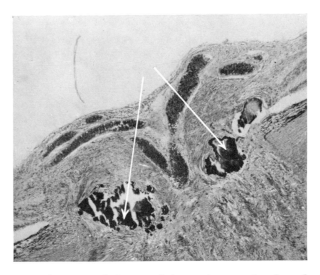

Figure 28. Another case of drusen of the optic nerve head producing a pseudopapilledema. Here a number of calcified bodies are present in the depth of the nerve head, pushing the nerve fibers up.

at his eyeground. He was then examined in our clinic. Vision in both eyes was better than 6/6. Visual fields were normal, and the pathologic findings were confined to the optic nerve heads. They appeared identical in both eyes.

The left optic nerve head shows an elevation of 4 diopters. The margins of the papilla are blurred. There were some retinal folds on the temporal side. The veins were perhaps slightly tortuous, but there were no hemorrhages or exudates. A spontaneous venous pulsation was visible.

The patient was seen by the Department of Neurology. No neurologic deficit was found. All laboratory tests, including electroencephalography, spinal fluid examinations, x-ray film of the skull, and air fillings remained normal. The patient was followed for over a year. The fundus picture did not change, and the patient remained in good health.

This case of pseudopapilledema cannot be differentiated from a true papilledema on a single examination. The appearance certainly resembles a true papilledema. A pseudopapilledema is frequently combined with a high hyperopia, but this was not the case in this young man. Only the negative results of all neurologic examinations and the prolonged follow-up allowed the diagnosis of a pseudopapilledema in this patient.

Macula I

Reel V-1. Drusen in macula

The right eye of a 52-year-old white man. The patient was hospitalized for a hyperventilation syndrome. Routine examination of the fundi revealed numerous small and large drusen in the macular area of both eyes. Vision in both eyes was 6/9.

The fundus of the right eye shows in and around the macular area numerous yellowish-white, punched-out lesions which lie deep to the retina. They are all sharply outlined, and some of them are surrounded by pigmentation. The retina itself is not involved.

Reel V-2. Central serous retinopathy

The right eye of a 22-year-old white female student. Three months before this photograph was taken, the patient complained of a loss of vision in the right eye. At that time, vision in the right eye was 6/12, and that in the left eye was 6/6.

The right macula shows a flat detachment. This area is approximately 4 discs in diameter. The fovea itself is depressed so that the typical cupid's bow appears. Small, yellowish-white deposits are seen in the retina. In the lower portion of this lesion is a flat pigmented area, deep to the retina. Another, similar, pigmented area is seen in the upper portion of the discoid macular lesion. A central scotoma corresponded to this macular edema. The patient was put on systemic steroid treatment, but the vision did not improve.

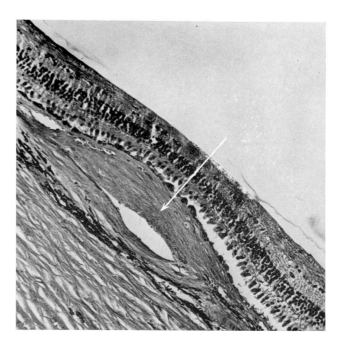

Figure 29. The usual senile drusen of the fundus have been illustrated in Figures 13 and 14. Similar drusen may, of course, occur in the macular area. This photomicrograph illustrates a larger accumulation of hyaline-like material between Bruch's membrane and the pigment epithelium in the macular area. The flow of nutrients from the choriocapillaris toward the neurosensory layer of the retina may be interfered with, and central visual acuity may suffer.

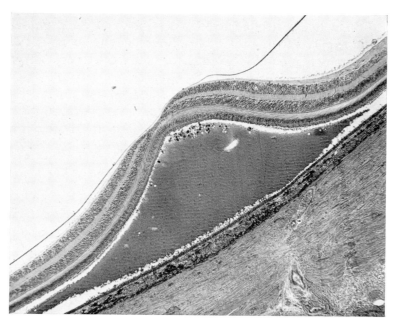

Figure 30. A central serous retinopathy is, in some instances, caused by a circumscribed retinal detachment in the macular area. This is illustrated on this photomicrograph. The macular area can be recognized by the thickening of the ganglion cell layer, the innermost nuclear layer (outside of the macula, this layer consists of only one row of nuclei). Below the retina is a stainable fluid, one of the hallmarks of an in vivo retinal detachment.

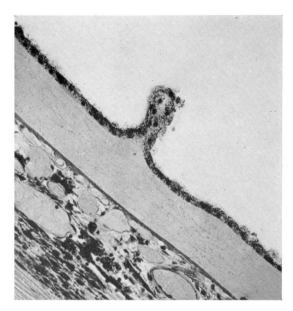

Figure 31. In other instances the central serous retinopathy is produced by a detachment of the pigment epithelium. This is the case in this eye in which the retinal pigment epithelium is detached from Bruch's membrane by an organizing protein-rich fluid. The eyes shown in Figures 30 and 31 were enucleated because of a clinical diagnosis of choroidal melanoma.

Reel V-3. Disciform macular degeneration

The left eye of a 41-year-old white male. The patient was referred to our clinic because of gradual loss of vision in both eyes. Vision in the left eye was reduced to 3/60 upon looking to the side. There was practically no central vision at all. Vision in the right eye was 6/6, and the right macula showed some scattered pigmentation.

The left macula illustrates a classical example of a disciform macular degeneration (Kuhnt-Junius degeneration). There is a slightly oval lesion in the macular area which is elevated and consists mainly of blood, connective tissue, and pigment. The center is a grayish-white, solid lesion which lies deep in the retina. This lesion is surrounded by deep hemorrhages. In addition, there are a few small hemorrhages on the central lesion and numerous yellowish-white deposits in the retina below and nasally. The central lesion itself shows beginning pigmentation. The retina is elevated and shows marked stress folds radiating from the foveal area toward the periphery.

The lesion may change in character because of fresh hemorrhages and progressive organization, and it may be difficult to differentiate such a senile macular lesion from a choroidal melanoma. The presence of blood in such lesions, however, speaks very much for a disciform macular degeneration, since small choroidal melanomas usually do not bleed. Furthermore, in many of these patients the lesion is bilateral, or at least some indication of a macular involvement can be found in the other eye. Finally, it has to be emphasized that in cases of doubt, the lesion should be observed. Since

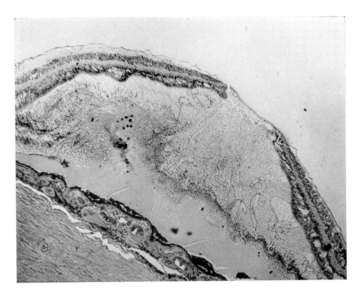

Figure 32. An early stage of a disciform macular degeneration. There is a circumscribed retinal detachment, but in this case the subretinal fluid is not only serous but also hemorrhagic. The blood makes the condition usually irreversible, and organization into a connective tissue scar will follow.

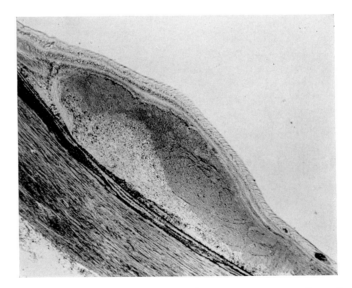

Figure 33. In this case of disciform macular degeneration the subretinal fluid is partly organized. The more superficial part of the subretinal space is occupied by blood. In the deeper layers connective tissue is present.

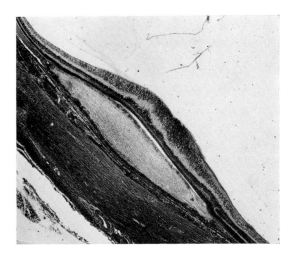

Figure 34. Typical connective tissue mound in the macular area which is so characteristic of disciform macular degeneration. Here, the connective tissue lies between pigment epithelium and retina.

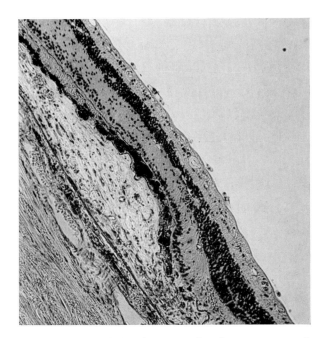

Figure 35. Another case of disciform macular degeneration under higher power than that shown in Figure 34. Here, most of the connective tissue lies between Bruch's membrane and the pigment epithelium. The tissue is quite dense but contains also a few vessels. The pigment epithelium is partly interrupted, partly hypertrophic.

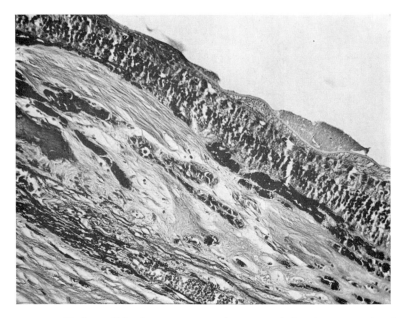

Figure 36. Under still higher power, another case of disciform macular degeneration shows the mound of connective tissue under the retina. Here, the pigment epithelium is absent in the center of the photomicrograph and is hypertrophic in the left upper corner. There are numerous defects in Bruch's membrane.

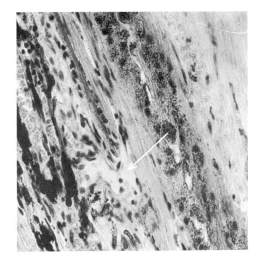

Figure 37. Disciform macular degeneration showing a very prominent break in Bruch's membrane through which a choroidal vessel sprouts into the subretinal tissue. These breaks in Bruch's membrane, with subsequent hemorrhages into the subretinal space, seem to be the first pathologic changes in this degenerative macular condition.

small choroidal melanomas usually have a good prognosis, there is no danger in watching such a lesion to see whether it develops into an unquestionable choroidal neoplasm or whether it remains a degenerative process of the macular area.

Reel V-4. Central chorioretinitis (histoplasmosis?)

The left fundus of a 35-year-old man. The patient had his first attack of poor vision in the left eye five years previously. At that time a central choroiditis was diagnosed. Several small, old areas of chorioretinal atrophy were found in both eyes at that time. He had a complete uveitis work-up, which was negative. Four years later he had a flare-up of the same lesion which quieted down after three months. Now again he suffers from an acute loss of vision in the left eye. The right eye had always been normal. When he came to our clinic, vision in the right eye was 6/3, and that in the left eye was 6/30.

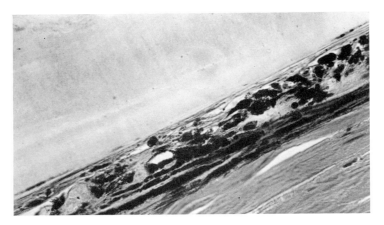

Figure 38. Specimen from an eye with old, atrophic, central chorioretinitis. In this area, choroid, pigment epithelium, and retina have fused to a dense scar tissue which appears heavily pigmented. Nothing is left of the original tissues.

The right macula is normal. In the periphery of the right fundus are numerous, punched-out areas of yellowish-white, chorioretinal atrophy. Similar areas are also present in the periphery of the left fundus. In the area of the left macula is an elevated, pigmented lesion 1½ discs in diameter. This lesion is not transparent and is gray-black in color. It is surrounded by a dense wreath of deep hemorrhages.

This again has been a case in which the differential diagnosis lies between a juvenile disciform macular degeneration and a central choroidoretinitis, perhaps due to histoplasmosis. In this case, the latter diagnosis seems to be more appropriate. The combination of such a macular lesion with peripheral, yellowish, punched-out areas is believed to be quite characteristic for histoplasmosis. The patient had a positive histoplasmosis skin test but a negative complement fixation test for *Histoplasma capsulatum.* The chest x-ray film was negative.

61

Reel V-5. Central chorioretinitis (histoplasmosis?)

The fundus of a 47-year-old white woman. Four to five months previously she noticed a blind spot in the right eye. Vision in the right eye was reduced to 6/60. The left eye was entirely normal, and vision remained 6/6.

The right eye shows a cystlike elevation just above the macula. This lesion is not entirely clear and has a grayish-white color. In it are a few deposits. A strand of grayish-white tissue extends like a tail from the cyst toward the lower nasal side.

The nature of this lesion remains in doubt. In the past, such macular elevations would have been called disciform degenerations. However, this does not quite fit the typical clinical picture and course of a Kuhnt-Junius degeneration. The patient is somewhat young for such a senile change, and the unilaterality of the condition also would speak against such a degenerative process. It should be emphasized that in recent years histoplasmosis has been thought to be an important etiologic factor in the production of such macular pseudotumors, and this patient had experienced a pulmonary histoplasmosis. On the other hand, such macular lesions have also been observed in patients with amebiasis. The patient's stool was examined repeatedly, but no amebae were found.

Reel V-6. Proliferative central chorioretinitis

This is the left fundus of a 24-year-old woman. The patient was aware of the fact that the vision in the left eye had been poor for many years. The right eye was entirely normal. Vision in the left eye was reduced to 6/60. The anterior segment was normal.

The left optic nerve head is pale. In the macular area is a very con-

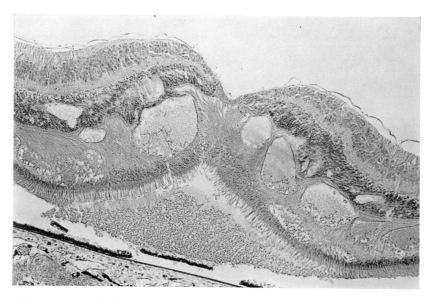

Figure 39. Marked cystoid degeneration of the macula together with a small circumscribed retinal detachment in that area. Here, the cystoid degeneration was due to a long-standing anterior uveitis.

spicuous elevated scar. This scar has a base of grayish-white tissue and a center of jet-black pigment. It is plainly visible that this scar stems from the choroid and elevates the retina. Small retinal vessels can be seen extending over it. Around the scar, especially in the lower nasal field, are numerous tension folds of the retina. The base of the scar is surrounded by a slight atrophy of the pigment epithelium and the choroid.

Two years earlier Hodgkin's disease was diagnosed in this patient. The diagnosis was made from a biopsy of a cervical lymph node. She received numerous series of radiation therapy and was later treated with chlorambucil, blood transfusions, and nitrogen mustard. Later on she was also treated by systemic prednisone. Her course was slowly but steadily downhill, and three months after this photograph was taken she died. The immediate cause of death was a cryptococcal meningoencephalitis. Although an intraocular involvement in Hodgkin's disease has been described, this macular lesion in the left eye seems to be independent of the patient's systemic disease. The cryptococcal infection was a terminal event and also could not have been the cause of the proliferative chorioretinitis.

Reel V-7. Macular cysts

This is the left eye of a 31-year-old white secretary. Since the age of 14 years, the patient was known to have diabetes mellitus, which was always difficult to control. She has been on insulin therapy ever since then. There is a strong family history of diabetes.

The patient was first seen in our clinic two years earlier with a marked diabetic retinopathy. Vision at that time was, with correction, 6/6 in both eyes. One year later she had a severe hemorrhage into the vitreous of the right eye, and vision was reduced to 6/60. When this photograph was taken, vision in the right eye was 6/15, with some haziness in the vitreous. Vision in the left eye was also 6/15, and this could not be improved.

Numerous microaneurysms can be seen in the left eye. The macular area is thickened and elevated. In its central part are small, lobulated cysts. There are three larger cysts present which seem to coalesce. They are surrounded by numerous retinal hemorrhages and a few deep exudates.

Macula II

Reel VI-1. Macular hole

The left fundus of a 60-year-old white woman. A cataract extraction had been performed on this eye one year previously. The vision in that eye had been good for nine months. From then on the patient experienced progressive painless loss of vision. There was never any pain or redness connected with this. Vision was reduced to 6/9 − 2 with correction. The right eye was also aphakic, and vision was with correction 6/6.

The right fundus was normal. The left macular area shows a round, reddish lesion which looks like a retinal hole. It cannot be decided whether this is a true hole or whether it is a cyst, the anterior wall of which could be extremely thin. This reddish area is somewhat elevated, and is surrounded by grayish reflexes in the retina. It does not lie exactly in the fovea but slightly nasal to it.

The patient has been observed for over two years, and the lesion has not changed, nor has the vision decreased.

Reel VI-2. Macular hole

The left eye of a 33-year-old white waitress. In the past, the patient had suffered from thyrotoxicosis. A thyroidectomy was performed nine years before she came to our clinic. This was repeated two years later for a toxic, nodular goiter. The patient received radioactive iodine ten years and one year previously. She was followed in the Thyroid Clinic.

One year ago she experienced a sudden loss of vision in the left eye. When she was first seen in our clinic, vision with correction in the right eye was 6/9, and that in the left eye was 6/60. The left macula showed a diffuse

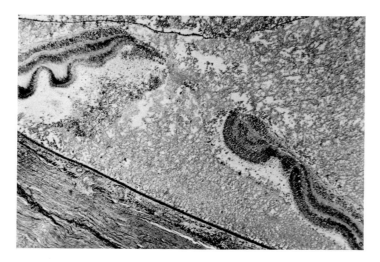

Figure 40. A macular hole. In this eye the hole was associated with a retinal detachment. There is an actual disruption of all the layers of the retina in the macular area.

edema. Most remarkable, however, was a sheathing of the retinal veins in both eyes. In addition, there were numerous newly formed retinal blood vessels, especially in the periphery. About one month later vision in the left eye was reduced to 3/60, and newly formed blood vessels were now also seen on the optic nerve head. Later on, hemorrhages and numerous cotton wool patches appeared in both fundi. Cells appeared in the vitreous, and two months later a large hole was visible in the left macular area.

The patient received a very thorough medical workup. Diabetes, infectious diseases, blood dyscrasias, and dysproteinemias could be excluded.

The eye condition went relentlessly downhill though the patient was intensively treated with steroids. Posterior synechiae appeared. Two years later vision in the right eye was 6/12, and that in the left eye was 1/60. The inflammatory signs in the anterior segment had disappeared, but the fundus picture did not change.

The stereoscopic picture shows, in high magnification, the macular area of the left eye. The oval retinal hole can be seen in the fovea. Through it a reddish reflex is visible. The entire macular area is edematous, and grayish reflexes are visible from the thickened retina.

Reel VI-3. Tension folds in macula

The left eye of a 40-year-old white man. The patient had noticed a progressive, painless loss of vision in this eye for nearly ten months. During the last month he also noticed a progressive protrusion of the eye. The right eye was entirely normal. The vision in the left eye was reduced to 2/60, which could, however, be improved to nearly 6/6 with a +6.00 lens. The left eye was markedly proptosed, and with the exophthalmometer a reading of 20 in the right eye and of 31 in the left eye was obtained. The left fundus showed a moderate amount of papilledema with no hemorrhages.

The photograph illustrates stress folds in the macular area. These folds are usually seen as horizontal lines crossing the macula. They are produced by pressure exerted on the posterior pole of the eye. They frequently indicate a tumor in the orbit or at least an increase in the contents of the orbit as in severe endocrine exophthalmos.

The visual field in the left eye revealed an enlarged blind spot. X-ray films of the skull and orbit were normal. Two weeks later the patient had an exploration of the left orbit by the Krönlein technique under general anesthesia. An elongated, bluish-red tumor was found in the muscle cone. It could be excised, and histologic examination revealed it to be a sclerosing hemangioma. The papilledema and the macular folds disappeared a few months after the operation.

Reel VI-4. Vitelline macular degeneration[*]

The right eye of a 7-year-old boy. The vision is 6/6 in both eyes. In both fundi the macular area is replaced by a round, yellowish, well-circumscribed mass. This mass seems to lie deep in the retina, and fine retinal vessels run over it. No obvious disturbance of retinal function accompanied this spectacular fundus picture.

This young boy presents the earliest stage of the so-called "hereditary vitelline macular degeneration." This is a familial disease, first described by Best in 1905. Ophthalmoscopic signs precede the symptoms by many years. Loss of central vision usually occurs in early adulthood, and progression is slow. The inheritance is usually autosomal dominant.

Reels VI-5 and VI-6. Vitelline macular degeneration[*]

The left eye of a 19-year-old college student. This patient is a member of the same family as the boy discussed in Reel VI-4. This young man had been under observation for more than a year, and because of loss of vision he had been on systemic steroid treatment off and on.

The first photograph (Reel VI-5) was taken when he noticed a rather abrupt loss of vision in the left eye. A deep intraretinal macular hemorrhage was seen which was surrounded by yellowish deposits. Visual acuity was 6/15. The patient was put on proteolytic enzyme for three days and again on a high dosage of systemic steroids.

After five weeks the vision in the left eye improved to 6/6 + 1.

The second picture (Reel VI-6) shows the fundus at this date. The hemorrhage has nearly absorbed but numerous small drusen-like areas are noted below and temporal to the main lesion.

Reel VI-7. Vitelline macular degeneration[*]

The right eye of a 42-year-old housewife. This patient is a member of the same family as the patients discussed in Reels VI-4 to VI-6. Visual acuity was 6/21 in the right and 6/30 in the left eye.

---

*From Braley, A. E., and Spivey, B. E.: Hereditary vitelline macular degeneration, Tr. Am. Ophth. Soc. **61**:339-368, 1963; published by University of Toronto Press.

In the right eye there is a dense, pigmentary hyperplasia in the form of a plaque situated in the macular area. This is surrounded by several yellowish deposits deep in the retina. The left macula, which is not illustrated, showed a circular area of depigmentation which was also surrounded by yellowish deposits.

This, then, is one of the appearances of an advanced or late case of vitelline macular degeneration. These late stages exhibit protean ophthalmoscopic pictures—in some eyes a hyperpigmentation and in other eyes a depigmentation of the macula dominates the ophthalmoscopic picture.

Systemic diseases I

Reel VII-1. Diabetic retinopathy

The left eye of a 61-year-old white man. The patient was found to have diabetes mellitus ten years previously. He was taking 35 units of insulin daily and was admitted to the hospital because of a hypoglycemic episode. When he came to our clinic, vision in both eyes was 6/9. The fundi in both eyes were quite similar.

Here, the left fundus shows some increase in the light reflexes on the arterioles. Around the macular area are numerous superficial hemorrhages and small microaneurysms which hang like berries on the vessels. The macula itself shows hyperpigmentation deep to the retina. Above and temporal from the macula are a number of deep, waxy exudates.

Reel VII-2. Severe diabetic retinopathy

The left eye of a 43-year-old white man. The patient had a history of diabetes for eight years. The disease has been under rather poor control. The patient had been twice previously admitted to the hospital because of acidosis. He was taking 70 units of insulin a day. He had experienced insulin shock about four or five times and he had repeated severe skin infections, diabetic neuropathy, and diabetic nephropathy.

For a year and a half before we saw him, vision became worse in both eyes. When he came first to our clinic, vision in the right eye was reduced to counting fingers at 3 feet and vision in the left eye was 6/60. The right eye showed a mixed injection and a diffuse corneal edema. There were cells in the anterior chamber, and the iris was covered with numerous newly formed blood vessels (rubeosis iridis). The fundus of the right eye could not be seen. The intraocular pressure in the right eye was 70 mm. Hg.

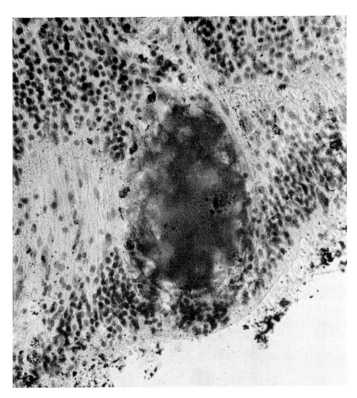

Figure 41. A very recent deep exudate in diabetic retinopathy. Sudan R was used to stain this section, and the deep deposit takes this neutral fat stain.

The left eye was externally normal, and the pressure in the left eye was 17 mm. Hg.

The left fundus shows a far-advanced diabetic retinopathy. The veins are markedly dilated. The arterioles are tortuous and show increased reflexes. There are numerous superficial hemorrhages especially temporal to the disc. There are also a number of microaneurysms present around the macular area. Most conspicuous are large, yellowish, fatty-looking deposits in the deeper part of the retina. These lie around the macular area and close to the disc.

The right eye soon became blind and had to be enucleated because of pain. The final diagnosis was absolute glaucoma due to diabetic rubeosis of the iris. Vision in the left eye remained stationary.

Reel VII-3. Severe diabetic retinopathy

The left fundus of a 60-year-old white man. A diagnosis of diabetes had been made in this patient twelve years previously, and he had been taking 40 units of insulin daily for eight years. Eight months before he came to our clinic, he experienced a rather sudden deterioration of vision in both eyes. This was more marked in the left eye. A change of glasses did not improve his vision. At the present he can read only with the help of a magnifying glass. It is noteworthy that his diabetes had always been under poor control.

Both fundi showed evidence of extensive and advanced diabetic retinopathy. The picture of the left fundus shows venous dilatation, numerous

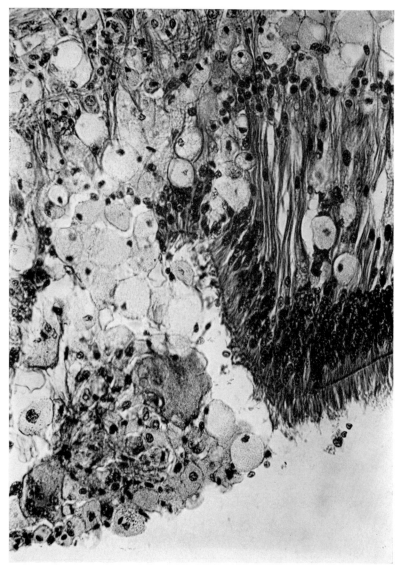

Figure 42. A later stage of a deep waxy exudate in diabetic retinopathy than that shown in Figure 41. In this case the fatty material has been engulfed and is phagocytized by numerous foam cells.

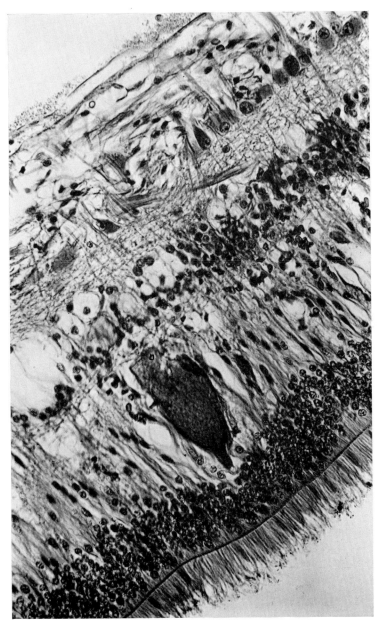

Figure 43. An even later stage of a deep waxy exudate in diabetic retinopathy than that shown in Figures 41 and 42. Here the material looks like hyalin and appears as an eosinophilic, amorphous deposit in the deep layers of the retina.

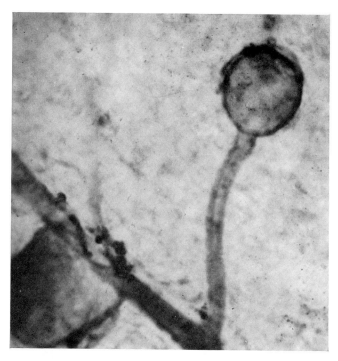

Figure 44. Flat section of the retina of a patient with severe diabetes. The section was stained with periodic acid-Schiff stain. The microaneurysms can be seen hanging like berries on the vascular tree.

superficial hemorrhages, and a few microaneurysms. There are also areas of cotton wool patches present. The biggest one is close to the disc in the 2 o'clock meridian. Both of these lie quite evidently in the superficial layers of the retina. In addition, there are a number of deep hemorrhages and numerous waxy, yellowish, exudates which lie in the deep layers of the retina, mainly on the temporal side. In the temporal lower periphery, a large yellowish deposit can be seen.

Urinalysis and kidney tests revealed a considerable degree of diabetic nephropathy. There was an early azotemia. The patient was put on a strict diet, and the insulin dosage was reduced to 30 units per day. On this program the blood sugar levels were fairly normal, and no sugar was spilled in the urine. The diabetic retinopathy did not change during the period of observation.

Reels VII-4, VII-5, and VII-6. Severe diabetic retinopathy with preretinal hemorrhage

The right eye of a 50-year-old white housewife. Diabetes had been diagnosed in this patient fourteen years previously, and she had been taking 70 units of insulin daily for two years. For a year before we saw her, she experienced tingling in the fingers, numbness of the left foot, and other symptoms of diabetic neuropathy.

Four months before she came to our clinic, she developed blurring of vision which was more marked in the left eye than in the right eye. When

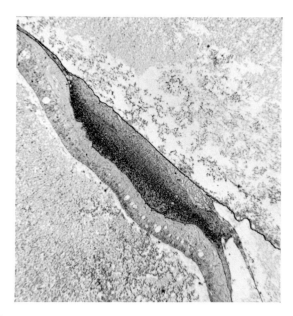

Figure 45. A detached retina in a patient with severe diabetic retinopathy There are two preretinal hemorrhages present. They lie between the internal limiting membrane and the vitreous body.

we examined her, vision in the right eye was reduced to 6/21 and that in the left eye to 6/60.

The first photograph (Reel VII-4) shows, under high magnification, the upper macular area of the right eye. Most impressive is the large number of microaneurysms. These can be seen not only on the venous side of the vascular tree, but also on the arteriolar side. In the deeper parts of the retina are numerous waxy, yellowish deposits. In the left lower corner is part of a preretinal hemorrhage.

The second picture (Reel VII-5) shows the area below the macula of the right eye. Most conspicuous here is the preretinal hemorrhage in the center of the photograph. In the deeper part of the retina are again numerous yellowish, waxy deposits, some of which coalesce to large areas. Another large hemorrhage can be seen in the right lower corner of the picture.

The third photograph (Reel VII-6) shows a more peripheral part of the right retina. There, again, is a large superficial hemorrhage and above it a smaller similar hemorrhage. The branches of the lower temporal vein show occlusion and sheathing with yellowish material. There are newly formed blood vessels on some branches of this vein. Again, in the deeper layers are numerous waxy deposits.

Reel VII-7. Severe diabetic retinopathy with preretinal hemorrhage

The right eye of a 23-year-old white man. The patient has had diabetes since the age of 7 years. At the present time he is taking 60 units insulin a day.

When he came to our clinic, he complained mainly about a brown line obscuring his vision on the right side. Vision in that eye had been poor for a number of years. His vision was 6/21 in the right eye and 6/9 in the left eye. Both eyegrounds exhibit severe diabetic retinopathy.

The right eye shows a preretinal hemorrhage below the disc. This hemorrhage obscures the lower temporal vein and artery. It has a nearly horizontal upper border. The veins are enlarged and show segmental constriction. The arterioles are definitely constricted, and some of them are occluded. This is especially true for the upper nasal artery, and in this area a fine mass of newly formed blood vessels lie in the superficial retina (rete mirabile). A similar condition can be seen near the lower artery. In addition, there are a number of small superficial hemorrhages below and nasal to the disc. The disc itself appears white and contains a number of sharply outlined, crystal-like structures, so-called drusen of the optic nerve head. Temporal to the disc are two small areas of deep chorioretinal atrophy.

Systemic diseases II

Reel VIII-1. Neovascularization in diabetic retinopathy

The left eye of a 79-year-old white woman. The patient had been treated for hypertension for eight years before we saw her and was known to have diabetes for four years. The blood pressure could be controlled quite readily with antihypertensive drugs. Six years before she came to our clinic she had an episode of an acute hemorrhage into the right vitreous. This cleared promptly. The diabetes was well controlled with diet and insulin.

When the patient was seen by us, vision with correction in the right eye was 6/15 and that in the left eye was 6/9. The fundus picture was nearly the same in both eyes. The retinal veins were tortuous and the arterioles attenuated. Numerous deep exudates and punctate hemorrhages were seen especially near the macula.

The fundus picture shows, under high magnification, newly formed blood vessels on the disc, forming a convolute at its upper margin. The retinal arterioles are constricted and show conspicuous crossing phenomena. In two areas the overlying arteriole compresses the underlying vein, and the thickened wall seems to interrupt the course of the vein. A few deep exudates can be seen nasal to the disc.

Reel VIII-2. Proliferating retinopathy in diabetes

The right eye of a 43-year-old white woman. The patient had had diabetes for at least twenty-seven years before she came to our clinic, and at the present she is on 30 units of insulin daily and 2 clorpropamide tablets a

75

day. The vision was slowly decreasing in the last years, especially in the right eye. When she came to us, vision in the right eye was reduced to 6/60, and that in the left eye was 6/9. The left fundus showed numerous deep exudates and hemorrhages together with a proliferating membrane in the temporal periphery.

The right fundus shows the classical picture of a proliferating retinopathy as it occurs in severe diabetes. In the vitreous a membrane of connective and glial tissue is present which contains numerous blood vessels sprouting out from the retina. This is the most severe stage of a diabetic retinopathy and will soon lead to a complete retinal detachment. The retina itself cannot be seen in this photograph, since the picture was focused on the membrane in the vitreous.

Reels VIII-3 and VIII-4. Hypertensive retinopathy

A 64-year-old white physician. The patient had been suffering from hypertensive cardiovascular disease for more than ten years. His vision had decreased three to four years before he came to us. When he was seen in our clinic, vision in both eyes was 6/21.

The right fundus (Reel VIII-3) shows marked vascular changes. The veins are tortuous and dilated. The arterioles are also tortuous and show a markedly increased light reflex of the vessel wall. The arterioles also show areas of localized attenuation. There are numerous cotton wool patches present, most of which are situated near or on an occluded arteriole. There are conspicuous crossing phenomena. Just below the disc is an arteriovenous

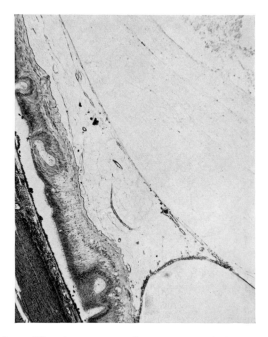

Figure 46. A proliferating retinopathy in severe diabetes. The retina itself is atrophic and folded. In front of it is a newly formed, vascularized connective tissue which stems mainly from blood vessels sprouting out from the retina. Contracture of this membrane will eventually lead to a retinal detachment.

crossing where the arteriole seems to interrupt the vein. The disc shows a temporal crescent of choroidal atrophy.

The left eye (Reel VIII-4) shows similar vascular changes. Again, there are numerous cotton wool patches in the superficial retina together with a few superficial and deep hemorrhages. Remarkable is an arterio-venous crossing above the macula where the arteriole has pushed the vein to one side. Most impressive are the numerous deep, yellowish deposits which surround the macular area, forming an incomplete star.

Reel VIII-5. Hypertensive retinopathy

The left eye of a 45-year-old white man who presumably had had a fairly recent onset of hypertension and renal disease. His blood pressure on admission was 238/144. The urine contained albumen with 20 white blood cells and an occasional red blood cell per high-power field. The BUN was 85 mg.%, and creatinine was 6.7 mg.%.

Both eyegrounds showed signs of advanced hypertensive retinopathy. The photograph shows the area above and temporal to the left disc. The veins are tortuous and widely dilated. The arterioles show localized constrictions. Most prominent are three areas of cotton wool patches in the center of the field. They are surrounded by superficial, flame-shaped hemorrhages. In the right lower corner of the picture are numerous deep, yellowish deposits which are arranged in lines, forming part of a macular star.

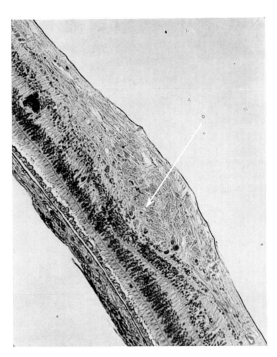

Figure 47. Histologic section of the retina from a severe hypersensitive retinopathy. The retina shows numerous deep deposits and in the center an accumulation of cytoid bodies. They lie characteristically in the nerve fiber layer and under this low magnification appear as a circumscribed swelling in this area.

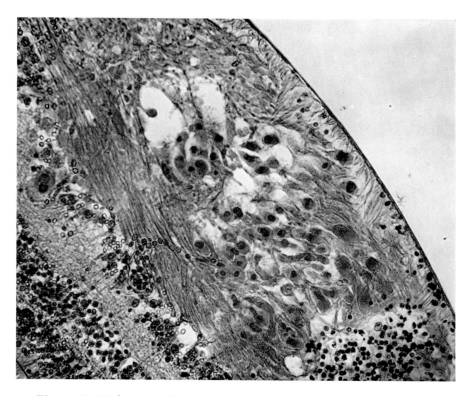

Figure 48. Higher magnification of an area of cytoid bodies. These structures do indeed resemble, to a certain extent, cells in the nerve fiber layer. Actually, they are the result of an anemic infarct in this area and correspond to the enlarged end bulbs of interrupted nerve fibers. There are a few red blood cells in the deeper layers of the retina.

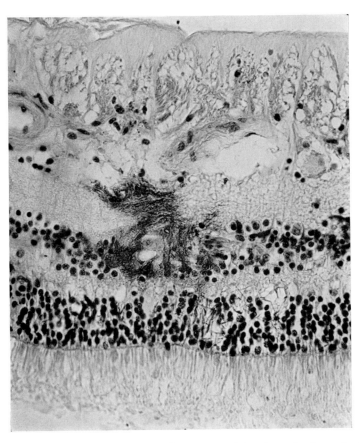

Figure 49. Edema in the retina with an area of inspissated edema in the center. This has led to destruction of some of the bipolar cells.

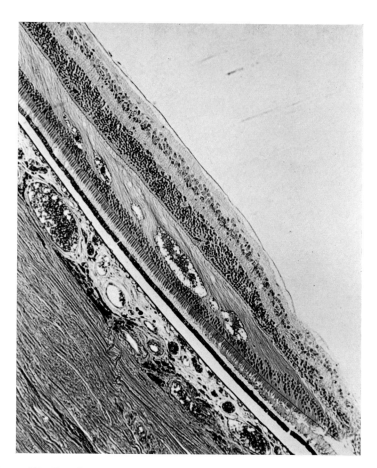

Figure 50. Histologic section through a macular star in hypertensive retinopathy. The fovea is in the right lower corner of the photomicrograph. Edema and deep deposits can be seen in the outer plexiform layer which, in the macular area, radiates away from the fovea and is called the Henle fiber layer. Deposits in this area will follow the radial direction of this fiber layer and, therefore, will assume a starlike figure.

Reels VIII-6 and VIII-7. Hypertensive retinopathy

A 55-year-old man. This patient was relatively well until about one year before these photographs were taken. At that time he woke up one night with an attack of difficulty in breathing and dizziness. He was hospitalized for two weeks and received oxygen. He was put on a reducing diet and lost about thirty-three pounds. The diagnosis at that time was hypertensive cardiovascular disease. Both his father and his mother had died from a stroke, and his brother suffers from heart disease. At that time his blood pressure was 230/150. The heart was slightly enlarged to percussion, and there was a soft systolic blow over the precordium.

When he was admitted to the Medical Department, a translumbar aortogram revealed a partial stenosis of the left renal artery and complete absence of the right renal artery. During a laparotomy the findings on the renal arteries were confirmed. At that time he also received a bifurcation graft of the abdominal aorta, since the aorta itself appeared to be 75% occluded. A bilateral lumbar sympathectomy was also carried out. The fundus photographs were taken one week before the operation.

The picture of the right eye (Reel VIII-6) shows an area temporal to and above the optic nerve head. The upper temporal artery has definitely increased reflexes and is somewhat tortuous. Where it crosses a venous branch, the underlying vein is displaced and appears markedly thin. Two branches from the artery can be observed running downward in the picture. The first branch is nearly completely occluded but still shows an interruption of the underlying vein. In this area are numerous superficial retinal hemorrhages. The second branch is markedly constricted and also compresses the underlying vein. Also, in this area are a few superficial hemorrhages.

The picture of the left eye (Reel VIII-7) shows the lower temporal artery and vein. The vein is markedly engorged. The artery is again tortuous and shows increased light reflexes. Again there are a number of marked arteriovenous crossing phenomena visible. Just above the center of the picture is a large superficial retinal hemorrhage surrounded by numerous smaller hemorrhages and whitish exudates. In the lower right of the picture are numerous newly formed venules and tortuous collaterals of the venous system.

After one year the blood pressure ranged between 190/105 in the supine position to 160/95 in a sitting position. All hemorrhages and exudates had disappeared from the fundi.

Systemic diseases III

Reel IX-1. Hypertensive retinopathy

The left eye of a 61-year-old white construction worker. Seven years ago, before this patient came to our clinic, he developed dizziness, and hypertensive cardiovascular disease was diagnosed. At that time his blood pressure was 180/120. When these photographs were taken, his blood pressure was 220/120. His blood pressure was labile but gradually responded to treatment.

The patient was followed in the Eye Clinic because of a chronic simple glaucoma. The intraocular pressure was 33 mm. Hg in both eyes. It could be well controlled with pilocarpine.

A photograph of the left eye shows a normal disc and conspicuously altered blood vessels. The arteries vary greatly in caliber, and there is marked localized constriction. The veins are engorged and tortuous. This is especially true of the nasal vein in the 3 o'clock meridian.

Reels IX-2 and IX-3. Hypertensive retinopathy

The left eye of a 50-year-old white widow. The patient had repeated kidney infections in the past. Her blood pressure was 145/90. She came to the hospital because of a left pyelonephritis. A biopsy of the left kidney showed completely sclerotic and hyalinized glomeruli. The tubules were largely replaced by a cronically inflamed, collagenous connective tissue. The small kidney arteries showed severe intimal thickening.

The first photograph (Reel IX-2) illustrates the posterior pole of the left eye. The retinal vessels show severe pathologic changes. The arterioles are tortuous, with localized constrictions. Some of the branches of the lower

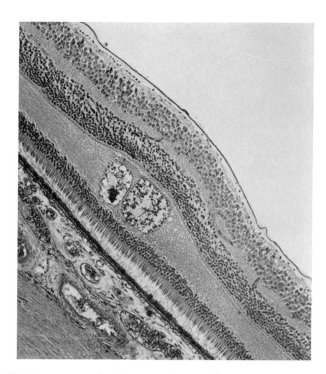

Figure 51. Severe retinal edema in the macular area. Two foci of inspissated edema are present in the outer plexiform layer.

temporal artery are invisible or are replaced by strands of whitish tissue (silver-wire arteries). The veins are tortuous. There are some newly formed blood vessels near the occluded vessels. There are marked arteriovenous crossing phenomena. The macula is depigmented, with some pigmentary hypertrophy above it (senile macular degeneration).

In the second picture (Reel IX-3) of the same eye, the area lateral to the macula is photographed. Here the silver-wire arterioles and occluded veins are even more conspicuous. The lower vein also shows sheathing. There are large, deep, yellowish exudates in the retina and also a number of superficial hemorrhages. Some of the vessels are apparently completely occluded.

Reel IX-4. Cholesterol plaque on arteriole

The right eye of a 64-year-old white woman. The patient was admitted to the Medical Department because of a five-month history of slowly progressive symptoms of congestive heart failure. She later developed acute pulmonary edema. The clinical diagnosis was mitral stenosis.

The eye findings were observed on a routine examination. The photograph shows a dilatation and tortuosity of the retinal veins. At the first branching of the upper nasal artery is a white-yellowish plaque partially obscuring the vessel. There is no definite occlusion, and the plaque seems to lie on the wall. There are definite arteriovenous crossing phenomena with depression of the underlying vein. This is best visible in the upper left corner of the picture. Nasally are some deep areas of choroidal atrophy.

83

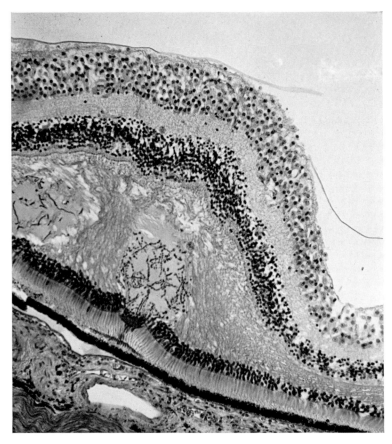

Figure 52. Another instance of severe macular edema in hypertensive retinopathy. In this patient, the edema has led to a folding of the retina.

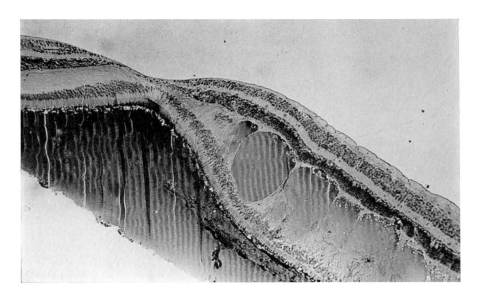

Figure 53. Extremely severe hypertensive retinopathy. The edema in the macular area is well visible. The outer plexiform layer is markedly thickened. The deposits of protein-rich fluid can be seen. In addition, there is a circumscribed detachment of the macular area.

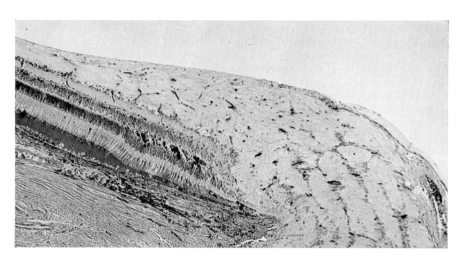

Figure 54. Another instance of severe hypertensive retinopathy. There is a papilledema present characterized by the elevation of the nerve fibers and the pushing aside of the retinal elements at the disc margin. In addition, deep hyaline-like deposits can be seen in the adjacent retina and a flat retinal detachment in the left corner of the picture.

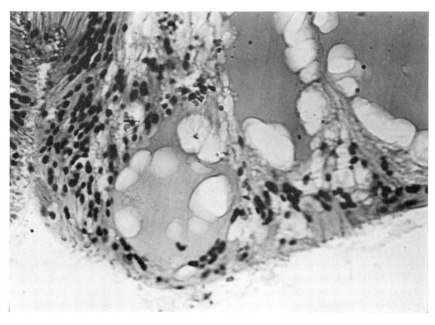

Figure 55. Severe retinal edema occurring in hypertension. This is a detached folded retina with partly serous, partly fatty deposits in the deepest layers.

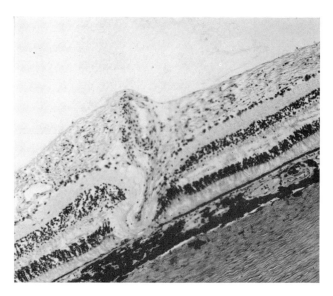

Figure 56. Cross section through an arteriovenous crossing in arteriolar sclerosis. The vein dips through all of the retinal layers and reaches the pigment epithelium. The overlying artery is thick-walled and elevates the internal limiting membrane.

Reel IX-5. Cholesterol plaque with arteriolar occlusion

The left eye of a 50-year-old white woman. One week before this patient came to our clinic, she experienced a sudden loss of vision in the lower half of the left visual field. There was no pain or redness connected with it. Her general health was good.

When she came to us, vision in the right eye was 6/9 and that in the left eye was 6/12. She had moderately large xanthelasmas on both upper eyelids. The eye findings, with the exception of the left fundus, were normal.

The fundus picture shows two glistening crystals, probably cholesterol, in one branch of the lower temporal artery. These lie below the macular area. The retina above the macula shows a diffuse, grayish-white discoloration and slight elevation. This retinal edema is due to an occlusion of a branch of the superior nasal artery. This occlusion was probably caused by a similar accumulation of shiny crystals. Corresponding to this arteriolar occlusion was a field defect in the left eye, nearly a complete inferior hemianopsia.

The patient was seen by the Medical Department. Her blood pressure was 130/84. Her serum optical density was elevated, and the serum cholesterol was high (330 to 354 mg.%). The patient was put on a low cholesterol diet. Treatment with anticoagulants was not thought to be indicated since the occlusion was one week old.

Reel IX-6. Cholesterol plaque with arteriolar occlusion

The right eye of a 69-year-old white housewife. At the age of 12 years, the patient had rheumatoid arthritis. Eleven years before we saw her she was hospitalized with the diagnosis of acute rheumatic fever. Since then she has been short of breath and tires easily. She was admitted to the Medical Department because of congestive heart failure.

During a routine eye examination, the occlusion of one branch of the lower temporal artery shown in the photograph was noticed. At the branching area lies a large glistening crystal. The original arteriole peripheral to the occlusion can be seen only faintly as a yellowish band. The blood flow now comes from the other branch of this arteriole and, by a tortuous anastomosis, enters again farther peripherally into the original arteriole.

Reel IX-7. Macroglobulinemia

The left eye of a 70-year-old white retired farmer. The patient was healthy all his life until a few months before we saw him when he experienced spells of dizziness, nausea, vomiting, and weakness. He was admitted to the Medical Department. An anemia of a normochromic and normocytic variety was detected. The serum globulins were markedly elevated (up to 10 to 11 gm.%). Many plasmacytes were found in the bone marrow. An ultracentrifugal analysis of the serum proteins revealed macroglobulins in concentration of 5,600 mg., compared with a normal value of about 200 mg. The patient was treated with testosterone and chlorambucil.

The photograph shows, in high magnification, the periphery of the left fundus. Plainly visible is the dilatation of the veins and their sausagelike constriction on the nasal side. There are also a few deep retinal hemorrhages present. The entire fundus looks pale. The picture is quite characteristic for macroglobulinemia.

Systemic diseases IV

Reel X-1. Anemia

The left eye of a 31-year-old white farmer. After a massive bleeding from the stomach, the patient was admitted to the Medical Service because of a secondary iron-deficiency anemia. On admission, his hemoglobin was 5.9 gm. with a hematocrit of 21%. The bone marrow revealed moderate erythroid hyperplasia with anisocytosis and hypochromasia.

The fundus is unusually pale. The arterioles are somewhat tortuous. In the 9 and in the 11 o'clock meridian close to the disc are two thin, superficial hemorrhages. These also show a white center which, in this patient, is due to the relative leukocytosis. The optic nerve head itself also appears pale.

The patient was given Imferon until the iron saturation was nearly 90%. The hemoglobin rose to 9 gm. with a hematocrit of 28%.

Reel X-2. Anemia

The right fundus of a 73-year-old white farmer. The patient came to the hospital because of severe anemia and congestive heart failure. His hemoglobin was reduced to 3.0 gm. with a hematocrit of 11%. The bone marrow was normal. Chromium-tagged red blood cell studies revealed a significantly shortened red blood cell survival time. A combined hypoplastic and hemolytic anemia was diagnosed, the etiology of which remained undetermined. The patient was treated with testosterone and numerous transfusions.

The fundus picture shows an unusually pale vessel tree. The color difference between the arterioles and the veins is reduced. The whole fundus lacks the yellowish background component which is, in part at least, due to the blood in the choroid. The small vessels, especially over the nerve head, are constricted and are hardly visible. In the periphery are numerous superficial flame-shaped retinal hemorrhages.

Reel X-3. Anemia with macular hemorrhage

The right fundus of a 19-year-old Negro student. One week before the patient came to us, he noticed loss of central vision in both eyes. There was no history of trauma.

This young man had had an anaplastic anemia diagnosed two years previously. He had received a total of more than thirty transfusions. He developed a secondary hemosiderosis. At the time when this macular hemorrhage occurred, the hemoglobin was 2.1 gm., the hematocrit was 8%, and the red blood cell count was 90,000. The white blood count was 6,850, with a normal differential count. The platelet count was 410,000, and no reticulocytes were seen in the peripheral blood.

Vision in the right eye was reduced to 6/21 and that in the left eye to 6/15. The left macula showed a brownish-grayish discoloration.

The right fundus shows a preretinal hemorrhage which has a horizontal fluid level. Above and temporal to the macula is another small retinal hemorrhage. The fundus shows not only the brownish coloration of a pigmented patient, but also the numerous light reflexes from the retina of a

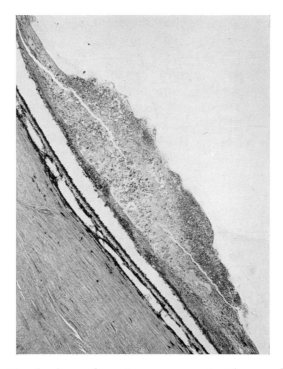

Figure 57. Macular hemorrhage in severe anemia. The macular area is nearly completely replaced by an extensive hemorrhage which has caused a central necrosis and thickening.

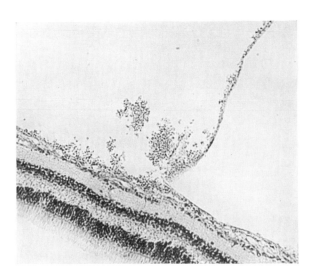

Figure 58. Superficial retinal and also subhyaloid hemorrhages in a patient with severe anemia.

young individual. This is most likely a spontaneous macular hemorrhage due to the anemia.

Reel X-4. Myelogenous leukemia

The right fundus of a 67-year-old white man. A chronic myelogenous leukemia had been diagnosed two years earlier. The patient was first treated with Myleran. Later he received x-ray therapy to the enlarged spleen. He was then given systemic steroids, and he also received numerous blood transfusions.

The white blood count rose from 20,000 to 50,000. The hemoglobin fell to 5.5 gm. and the hematocrit to 19%.

The fundus shows hyperemic veins and numerous superficial retinal hemorrhages. These hemorrhages have a feathery appearance as they lie superficially in the nerve fiber layer. They have a whitish center, so characteristic for a relative or absolute leukocytosis.

The patient developed a secondary hemolytic anemia and died three months later. The autopsy confirmed the diagnosis of chronic myelogenous leukemia with involvement of the liver, spleen, and lymph nodes.

Reel X-5. Myelogenous leukemia

The left eye of a 24-year-old white man. The patient became ill only seven weeks before his admission to the hospital. He came down with fever, sore throat, and swelling of some lymph nodes. When he was admitted, his hemoglobin was 9.2 gm., red blood cell count was 2.84 million, white blood cell count was 91,025, and hematocrit was 27%. The differential count of the white blood cells in the peripheral blood showed 91% blasts. The bone marrow showed 78% blasts, some of which appeared to be taking on fine granulations. The patient was treated with 6-mercaptopurine and prednisone.

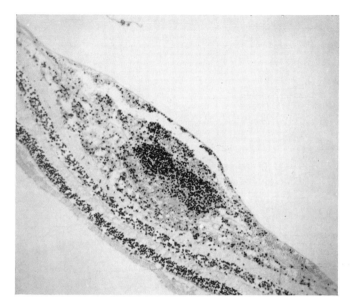

Figure 59. Extensive superficial hemorrhage in a patient who died from leukemia. The white center of the hemorrhage is due to a concentration of leukocytes.

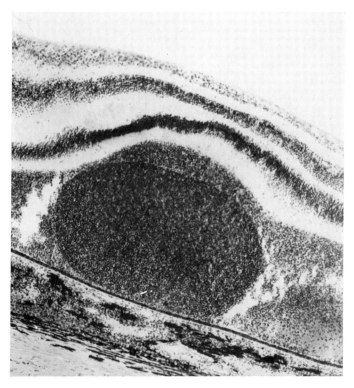

Figure 60. Extensive subretinal hemorrhage in a patient with severe leukemia. **91**

When the patient was seen in our clinic, vision in the right eye was 6/12 and that in the left eye was 6/6. There were numerous hemorrhages in both eye grounds. The fundus picture shows, in high magnification, the left disc with two adjacent, superficial retinal hemorrhages. The one in the 2 o'clock meridian has a small white center characteristic for leukemia. The veins are somewhat engorged. The disc itself shows a deep, but physiologic, cup.

The patient died one month later. The diagnosis was acute myelocytic leukemia.

Reel X-6. Chloroquine retinopathy

The left eye of a 51-year-old white woman. This patient started having joint pain from rheumatoid arthritis six years before we saw her. She was given 750 mg. of chloroquine per day. The joint pain soon improved, and the dose was gradually reduced to 250 mg. per day. She had been on this reduced dosage for three years when she came to our clinic. On this medication the joint symptoms have been well controlled, but there has been a progressive loss of vision in both eyes.

When the patient was seen in our clinic, vision in both eyes was reduced to 6/15. The anterior segments were normal. The visual fields showed large cecocentral scotomas. The fundus picture was the same in both eyes. The left macular area is illustrated in the photograph shown here. In the macular area is a central disc of dark pigmentation. The pigment lies deep in the retina and is fluffy. This is surrounded by a clear reddish

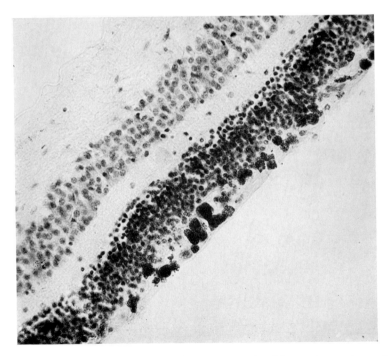

Figure 61. A histologic section of an eye with chloroquine retinopathy. The ganglion cells are rarefied. A dark, black pigmentation is visible in the outermost layers of the retina.

zone which is limited by another wreath of deep grayish pigmentation.

The fundus picture is quite characteristic for this type of toxic retinopathy. In more advanced cases the pigmentation may extend farther into the periphery.

The drug was discontinued, but neither the loss of vision nor the fundus changes showed any improvement.

Reel X-7. Mellaril retinopathy

The left fundus of a 23-year-old white student. A few months before we saw this patient he had been hospitalized because of an attack of acute schizophrenic psychosis. He was given tranquilizers and later received nine electroshock treatments. After this he was given a phenothiazine derivative, thioridazine. He received a maximum dose of 1,400 mg. daily, which after a month was reduced to 1,000 mg. daily. On the fifty-sixth day of treatment with this drug, the patient first complained of loss of vision. At that time he was receiving 800 mg. daily.

When he was first seen in our clinic, vision in the right eye was reduced to 6/9 + 3 and that in the left eye to 6/6 − 1. There were slight pigmentary changes in both macular areas. The eyes were otherwise normal. The drug was discontinued after he had received a total dose of approximately 50 to 60 Gm. He was switched to another phenothiazine derivative.

The patient was followed very carefully. The visual fields showed a moderate but definite constriction. The dark adaptation curve was quite abnormal and definitely flattened. Four weeks later definite pigmentation developed in the macular area.

The visual functions slowly improved with the withdrawal of the drug. Two months after the withdrawal, the central vision had improved to 6/6 in both eyes and the visual fields were nearly normal. The dark adaptation curve also was almost normal.

The pigmentation in the macular areas has, however, not changed very much. The photograph shows the granular pigmentation in the deeper parts of the retina in and around the macula. In the fovea itself is an area of dark redness. The pigmentation extends into the periphery but becomes less and less marked and dense.

Toxic retinopathies have been observed with certain phenothiazine derivatives. Some of them had to be withdrawn because of the high incidence of ocular side effects. Thioridazine apparently gives rise to a toxic retinopathy only when given in a daily dosage of more than 1,400 mg. for a prolonged period of time.

Vascular changes

Reel XI-1. Occlusion of central retinal vein

The right eye of a 72-year-old woman. The patient experienced a sudden, nearly complete loss of vision in the right eye two days before she came to our clinic. Vision in that eye was reduced to light perception and correct projection. Vision in the left eye was 6/9 + 2, and the only positive findings on that side were some arteriosclerotic changes in the retinal vessels. The patient had a slightly increased blood pressure but was otherwise in good condition.

The photograph of the right fundus shows, in the center, the blurred optic nerve head. Extending from it are numerous extensive superficial hemorrhages which cover nearly all the structures of the retina. Only farther out in the periphery can dilated and tortuous veins be seen. The retinal hemorrhages decrease in intensity toward the periphery but are still present in the area of the equator.

The patient was treated with anticoagulants for a few weeks, but the condition in the right eye did not improve. Nearly three months later the patient developed a secondary glaucoma which eventually led to an enucleation of that globe. Such severe glaucomas occur after a few months in about one-third of the eyes with central vein occlusion.

Reel XI-2. Occlusion of central retinal artery

The right eye of a 63-year-old man. This patient lost the vision in his right eye quite suddenly four days before he came to us. Before that, vision in that eye had been good although he had had a transient visual loss

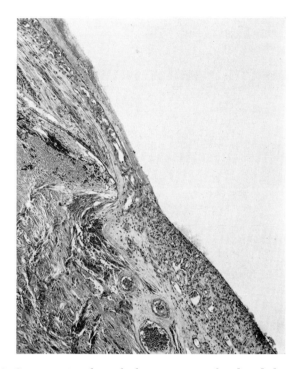

Figure 62. Cross section through the optic nerve head and the adjacent retina in a case of old central vein occlusion. The central vein itself is not visible anymore, but there are numerous new-formed blood vessels on the cribriform plate and in front of it.

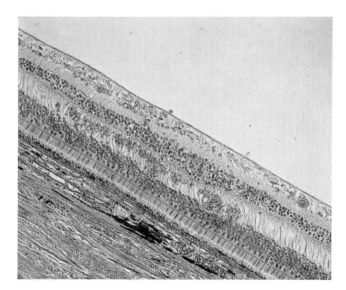

Figure 63. Cross section through a retina in a case of a fairly recent central vein occlusion. Hemorrhages are present in all the layers of the retina.

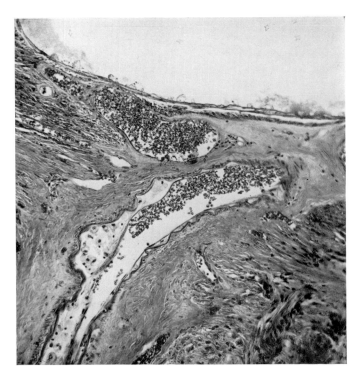

Figure 64. Cross section of the optic nerve head. The central retinal artery is in the center and shows thickened walls with conspicuous subintimal thickening. This has led to an occlusion of the artery in the lower part of the photomicrograph.

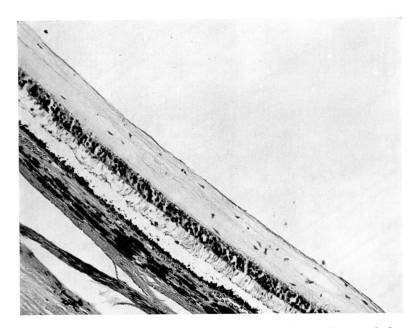

Figure 65. Anemic infarct of the retina due to the occlusion of the central retinal artery. The inner layers of the retina are necrotic. The outer layers, especially the rods and cones which derive their blood supply by diffusion from the choriocapillaries, are not affected.

three years before. The latter cleared up within an hour. His general health was apparently good, although he complained of heart trouble.

The left eye was essentially normal with a vision of 6/6. The retinal arterioles on that side showed increased light reflexes and tortuosity.

The right eye had a vision of light perception only, and the pathologic changes were confined to the fundus.

The photograph of the right fundus shows a marked retinal edema especially around the macula. The retinal arterioles are extremely thin. There are a few superficial vessels on the temporal side of the disc. The retinal edema causes a grayish discoloration and elevation of the retina at the posterior pole. In the upper left corner of the picture are two cotton wool patches. The fovea itself shows the characteristic cherry-red spot. This is a contrast phenomenon which is due to the fact that in the fovea the retina is so thin that the edema does not amount to much. In that area the red choroid still shines through, which is in contrast to the adjacent retina, which, because of the intensive edema, has become opaque. Vision in the right eye was not recovered.

Reel XI-3. Occlusion of retinal arteriole

The right eye of a 20-year-old salesman. Twenty-four hours before admission, the patient noticed a blurred spot in the right eye. He denied any trauma or infection. At the age of 4 years he had suffered from rheumatoid heart disease.

When he was seen in our clinic, vision in the right eye was reduced to

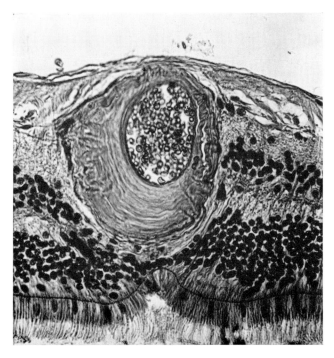

Figure 66. Cross section through the retina shows a very marked arteriolar sclerosis. The media of this arteriole is conspicuously thickened.

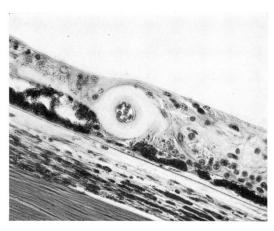

Figure 67. Cross section of the retina illustrating another example of arteriolar sclerosis. This section is from the periphery of the retina, and atrophy of the retinal layers accompanies this vascular disorder.

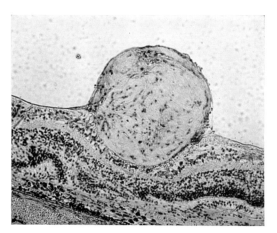

Figure 68. Complete occlusion of a thick-walled retinal arteriole. Here the lumen is replaced by proliferating connective tissue. The vessel is elevated above the level of the internal limiting membrane.

6/12. The left eye was entirely normal, and vision in that eye was 6/4.5. The visual field of the right eye showed a defect for small targets below the midline.

The photograph of the right fundus shows part of the retinal edema which was visible temporal to and above the disc. The outlines of the disc can be seen in the right lower corner of the picture. The upper temporal artery had a yellowish plaque on the disc. In the lower half of the photograph may be seen the edematous retina which appears gray and opaque. At the border of the opaque and the clear retina are a few cotton wool patches and numerous retinal folds.

Note: The stereoscopic effect is limited because of the inability to dilate the pupil widely for adequate parallax.

Reel XI-4. Occlusion of retinal vessels

The left eye of a 66-year-old white widow. The patient had had diabetes for nine years. It was well controlled with Orinase and diet. She was referred to our hospital because of a gangrenous ulcer at the base of the great toe of the right foot.

On admission no pulsation was palpated below the femoral artery on the right side. Blood pressure was 145/85. The fundus on the right side showed tortuous arterioles with marked arteriovenous nicking.

The left fundus shows an old occlusion of the upper temporal vessels. The artery is threadlike near the disc, and in the area of the first branching the vessel wall is markedly thickened. From that area peripherally, white strands replace the arteries and the veins.

The right foot had to be amputated above the knee, and the final diagnosis was severe, systemic arteriosclerosis with diabetes.

Note: The meniscus of light at the left side of the photograph is a catoptric image.

Reel XI-5. Occlusion of retinal vessels with neovascularization

The right eye of a 54-year-old white man. The patient had hypertensive cardiovascular disease and severe diabetes. Vision in the right eye was reduced to 6/21 and that in the left eye to 6/30.

The photograph of the right fundus illustrates occlusive vascular phenomena, as can be seen in severe hypertensive retinopathies, and neovascularization in the retina, as can be seen in severe diabetic retinopathy. The upper temporal artery is closed about 2 disc diameters away from the papilla and ends there abruptly in a tree of small, newly formed blood vessels which lie superficially in the retina. The corresponding vein is also interrupted, and the main branch is replaced by a yellow, grayish band. A number of collaterals have been established. There are also a few superficial retinal hemorrhages. Temporal and adjacent to the disc there are also some newly formed vessels sprouting into the superficial layer of the retina.

Reel XI-6. Telangiectasia of retinal vessels

The left eye of a 13-year-old girl. Vision in both eyes was 6/6. The right was absolutely normal.

The left disc shows on its margin a number of dilated new-formed blood vessels. They are mainly on the nasal and upper margin. A few may also be seen temporally. There is a small but deep physiologic excavation and a definite crescent of choroidal atrophy of the temporal side. The condition did not change over a period of two years' observation.

Note: The whitish ghost-like disc beyond the retina in the left center of the picture is a photographic artifact from a dust spot on the camera lens.

Reel XI-7. Choroidal sclerosis

The left eye of a 47-year-old housewife who has had night blindness for many years. For six to eight years before she came to our clinic, her vision has decreased even when the illumination is good. She knows that one of her sisters and one of her brothers are affected with the same visual difficulty.

At present, vision in both eyes is reduced to 6/30. The anterior segments are normal.

The visual fields on both sides are markedly, but irregularly, constricted. The electroretinogram is abolished to the usual stimuli. The dark adaptation curve is flattened and consists only of her defective cone response.

The photograph shows the atrophy of the retinal pigment epithelium with some pigment changes in the retina. The choroidal vessels appear as a network of yellowish-white, sharply outlined, broad lines.

Chorioretinitis

Reel XII-1. Active juxtapapillary chorioretinitis

The left fundus of a 24-year-old white carpenter. Two weeks previously the patient noticed some loss of vision in the left eye. This occurred quite suddenly.

When he first came to our clinic, the right eye was entirely normal, and vision in that eye was 6/5. The anterior segment of the left eye was normal, and vision in that eye varied between 6/12 and 6/9. In the beginning the disc was diffusely blurred and the veins were engorged. There were a few hemorrhages on the disc. After a few days during which the patient was on intensive steroid treatment, the diffuse blurriness of the disc disappeared and a localized lesion next to the disc became apparent.

The fundus photograph shows the acute chorioretinitis next to the disc in the 2 o'clock meridian. This is a yellowish-white dense mass which bulges the retina forward. It is indistinct in its outlines and is surrounded by a rim of dark pigmentation. The disc has still somewhat blurred margins, and the vessels are hyperemic. Downward and outward from the lesions can be seen numerous tension folds in the retina. After a few months this active lesion turned into an area of juxtapapillary chorioretinal atrophy. Treatment consisted of systemic steroids. Vision improved to 6/6 + 3.

Reel XII-2. Old juxtapapillary chorioretinitis

The left fundus of a 22-year-old white student. The patient had her first attack of decreased vision two and a half years before she came to our clinic. At that time she was treated with systemic steroids, and her **101** vision improved. About three months before we saw her, she again noticed decreased vision, more in the left eye than in the right.

When she was first seen by us, vision in the right eye was 6/21 and that in the left eye was 6/60. At that time the patient was two months' pregnant.

The right fundus shows a number of small areas of chorioretinal atrophy. These extend from the disc especially above and temporally. In these areas the choroidal vessels can be seen. Above the disc are also some areas of depigmentation. Toward the macula there are large areas of depigmentation.

The patient received a uveitis workup, but no etiologic factor could be found. There was slight improvement following systemic steroid treatment.

Reel XII-3. Acute peripheral chorioretinitis

The left fundus of an 18-year-old student. Two years previously the patient had an episode of inflammation and redness of the left eye. Since then, vision in the left eye has been reduced. The right eye was always normal. At the time he came to our clinic, vision in the right eye was 6/5 and that in the left eye was 6/12.

The left anterior segment is normal. There are fine pigmented particles in the left vitreous. In the left periphery near the equator is an oval, elevated, yellowish-white lesion. The periphery of this lesion shows beginning choroidal atrophy. The center of the lesion is grayish-white. Next to the lesion are some deep hemorrhages.

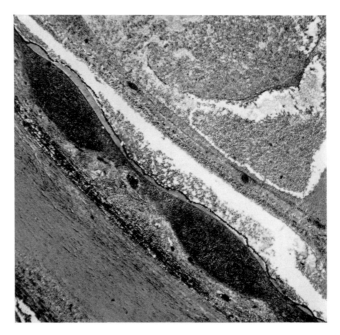

Figure 69. Severe acute choroiditis. There are two large areas of inflammatory infiltrates in the choroid. In addition, there is a retinal detachment, and inflammatory cells are also present in the vitreous.

The uveitis workup was essentially negative. Skin tests, x-ray films of the paranasal sinuses and hands, and serologic tests all were negative. The methylene-blue dye toxoplasmosis test was positive in dilution of 1:32. The diagnosis of toxoplasmosis was entertained. It was also thought possible that the patient was suffering from an infestation with *Toxocara canis*. His skin test, however, did not substantiate this. The patient improved following systemic steroid treatment, and within two months vision had been restored to 6/6.

Reel XII-4. Old peripheral chorioretinitis

The left fundus of a 39-year-old white physician. The patient experienced an attack of choroiditis in the left eye five years previously. Since then he had been bothered by vitreous opacities in that eye. The vision in both eyes was 6/5, and the right eye was entirely normal. The left vitreous showed a marked detachment and presenile vitreous changes. Numerous old vitreoretinal adhesions were present.

In the nasal periphery of the left eye near the equator is an old chorioretinal scar. This appears as a flat, heavily pigmented, discrete lesion with areas of chorioretinal atrophy around the edge. Within the margin of hyperpigmentation are numerous punched-out, yellowish areas of atrophy. The

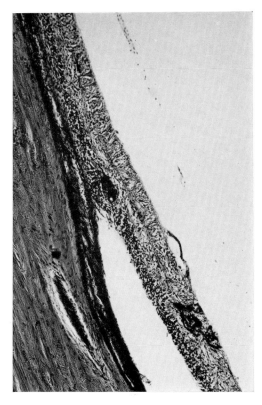

Figure 70. Cross section through an eye with an old disseminated chorioretinitis. In the upper part of the photomicrograph are dense chorioretinal adhesions. The retina itself is atrophic and shows numerous areas of pigment accumulation. In the area of chorioretinal adhesion, the pigment epithelium is absent.

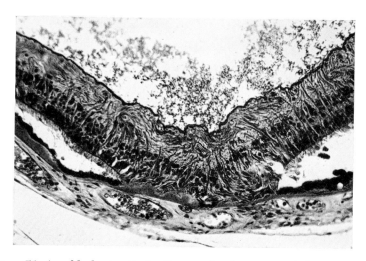

Figure 71. An old chorioretinal adhesion. In the center of the photomicrograph, choroid and retina are fused together. In this area the pigment epithelium is absent, but there is marked hypertrophy of this layer adjacent to the scar. The chorioretinal adhesion is accentuated here because of the artifactitious retinal detachment around it.

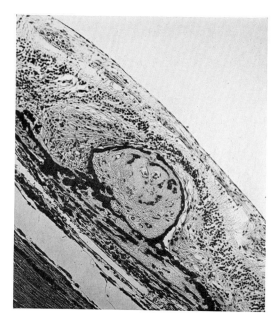

Figure 72. Area of hypertrophic chorioretinal scarring. There is proliferation of the pigment epithelium and of connective tissue. The retina is atrophic.

choroidal vasculature shines through the central part of the scar. The retinal vessel crossing this scar is slightly elevated.

Note: The two small, gray, flattened oval shapes in the center of the picture are photographic artifacts due to reflections in the camera lens. The picture is oriented so that the top edge is toward the nasal periphery.

Reel XII-5. Acute central chorioretinitis (toxoplasmosis?)

The left eye of a 37-year-old white housewife. Four weeks before the patient came to our clinic, she noticed a loss of vision in the left eye. She had always enjoyed good health. When she was first seen, vision in the right eye was 6/6 and that in the left eye was 6/24. The right eye was entirely normal. The left anterior segment was normal.

The left disc is surrounded by a pigment ring and some choroidal atrophy. Somewhat below the left macular area is a circumscribed retinal edema. Here, the retina is definitely elevated. This edema is circular and about 1½ disc diameters in size. Near the lower edge of this edema is an area of retinal pigmentation of nearly jet-black color. This is surrounded by some whitish-yellow exudation into the deep retina. Similar material is present in the center of the edema, surrounded by a half circle of a deep hemorrhage.

The uveitis workup was essentially negative. The only positive finding was a 1:64 positive toxoplasmosis dye test. The patient was treated with Daraprim, sulfadiazine, and systemic steroids. The toxoplasmosis dye test remained positive for about two months. The retinal edema decreased

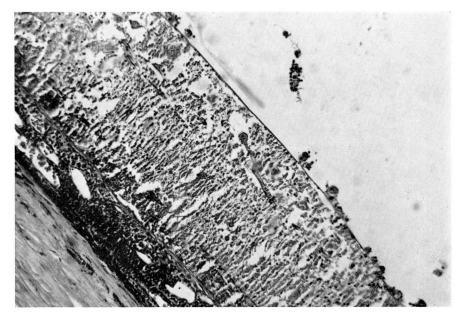

Figure 73. Toxoplasmosis chorioretinitis. The inflammatory cells are still visible in the choroid. There is marked necrosis in the retina. It is in this area that the protozoon can be found.

105

under treatment, and the yellowish exudates slowly disappeared. After three months, vision in the left eye with correction was nearly 6/6.

Reel XII-6. Central chorioretinal scar

The right fundus of a 30-year-old housewife. Five years previously she had her first attack of loss of vision in the right eye. At that time a central chorioretinitis was diagnosed, and she had been treated with systemic steroids. The vision improved considerably, but three weeks before she was seen in our clinic she had a recurrence of this loss of vision in one eye.

When she was seen by us, vision in the right eye was reduced to light perception with correct projection. The left eye had always been normal, and vision in that eye was 6/6. The right eye showed a ciliary injection, and numerous mutton-fat precipitates were present on the posterior corneal surface. The anterior chamber showed a flare with very few cells in the aqueous. The pupil was bound down to the lens with two synechiae.

The right disc shows a certain pallor of the temporal half. There is a marked temporal crescent, and temporal to that is an area of choroidal atrophy. Most conspicuous, however, is a macular lesion which consists of a dark retinal mass that lies directly in the center of the macula and is surrounded by a margin of pigmentation. The area has the shape of a pear, and above and nasal to it are some additional areas of retinal pigmentation. This mass lies deep in the retina, and one vessel from below crosses over it. Deep to this retinal mass is a much larger area of choroidal atrophy. In the

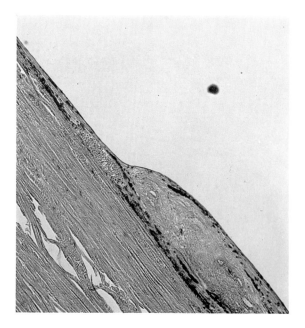

Figure 74. Cross section through a hypertrophic, central chorioretinal scar. In the upper part of the photomicrograph is an area of extreme atrophy. Here, choroid and retina are replaced by a thin band of connective tissue. In the lower part of the photomicrograph there is proliferation of the connective tissue and of pigment-bearing cells. The retina itself has disappeared.

periphery of this area some of the choroidal vessels can be seen. At the lower edge of the choroidal atrophy is some deep pigmentation.

Not visible on the fundus photograph is another chorioretinal lesion which was regarded as a satellite lesion and was present in the inferior periphery. The patient had a large central scotoma. The only positive skin test was the one for toxoplasmosis. The toxoplasmosis dye test was positive in a dilution of 1:64. The patient received a course of chemotherapy for toxoplasmosis, but the vision did not improve beyond 2/60.

Reel XII-7. Disseminate chorioretinitis

The right fundus of a 37-year-old white housewife. The patient had noticed a blurring of vision in the right eye one year before she came to our clinic. Soon thereafter she noticed also a decrease of vision in the left eye. This was connected with metamorphopsia. When she was first seen by us, vision in the right eye was 6/5 and that in the left eye was 3/60. The anterior segments were normal in both eyes. The left eye revealed an active central chorioretinitis. Although the patient had a thorough workup for uveitis, the etiology of this inflammation could not be determined.

On the right side numerous chorioretinal scars are visible. Most pronounced are areas of chorioretinal atrophy surrounding the disc. Next to the disc is another small area of choroidal atrophy which is just temporal to and below the macula. Other such areas can be found in the periphery of the fundus, but the macula in the right eye is not involved.

Tumors

Reel XIII-1. Choroidal nevus

The right fundus of a 49-year-old white woman. The lesion was found incidentally when the patient came in for a change of her reading glasses. Vision was 6/6 in both eyes.

Below and temporal from the disc is a slate-gray lesion. It is about 2 disc diameters in size and is slightly oval. It lies deep to the retina, and the retinal vessels course over it undisturbed. The lesion is not elevated, nor does it cause any scotoma.

Reel XIII-2. Choroidal nevus

The left eye of a 47-year-old white woman. Vision in both eyes was 6/6.

Along and under the inferior nasal artery is an accumulation of slate-gray deep pigment. In the pigmented area are numerous white, sharply outlined foci. The lesion is certainly beneath the retina but seems to be elevated at least on one side, where the inferior nasal artery shows a definite hump. The slate-gray color and the presence of numerous drusen are quite characteristic for a choroidal nevus.

Reel XIII-3. Nevus of pigment epithelium

The left fundus of a 63-year-old white woman. This dark pigmented lesion in the nasal part of the fundus was an incidental finding during an

108

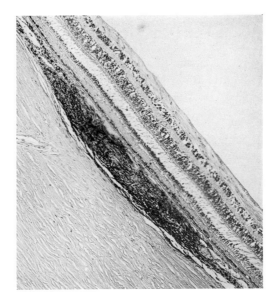

Figure 75. An accumulation of choroidal melanocytes in a well-circumscribed area of choroidal nevus. The degree of pigmentation may vary. The tumor does not enlarge the choroid or elevate the retina. It does not involve the choriocapillaris, and there is no damage to the overlying retinal tissue. The cells are of uniform character and there is hardly any mitotic activity.

examination and refraction. Vision in both eyes with correction was 6/6.

The pigmented area is flat and sharply outlined and lies under the retina. It is jet-black in color and has not changed in size during the period of observation.

Reel XIII-4. Choroidal melanoma

The left fundus of a 41-year-old white housewife. When the patient came in for a refraction, it was noted that the left eye had a vision of only 3/60. Four years previously vision in that eye had been 6/6. The anterior segment of the left eye was normal. The right eye was entirely normal, and vision on that side was 6/5.

The neoplasm can be distinctly seen in the area of the left macula. The optic nerve head, which lies to the left of the photograph, is not involved. The tumor is surrounded by a ring of dark pigmentation. Temporal to it is a conspicuous solid retinal detachment. The neoplasm itself is only slightly pigmented in the center. The temporal and upper margin of the tumor cannot be seen. In the retina are small yellowish deposits which are especially clearly visible in the lower nasal periphery of the tumor. The retinal vessels cross over the choroidal neoplasm without being affected but are markedly elevated.

Histologic examination of the enucleated left globe revealed a melanoma of the choroid of the epithelioid type (Path. #5256), and the photomicrograph of the eye is illustrated in Figure 76.

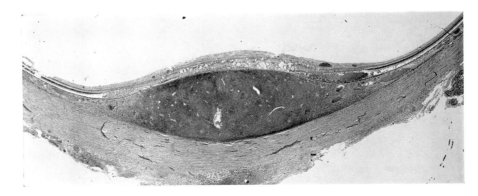

Figure 76. A small melanoma at the posterior pole of the enucleated globe. The choroid is definitely thickened, and the retina over it shows cystoid degeneration. There is also a slight retinal detachment along the slopes of the tumor.

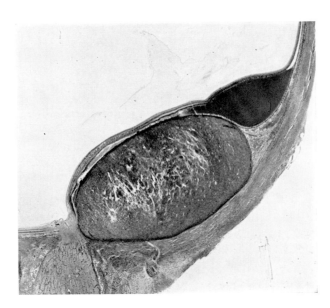

Figure 77. A melanoma adjacent to the optic nerve head. The tumor is still confined within the thickened choroidal tissue and has not yet broken through Bruch's membrane. The retinal detachment at the periphery of the tumor is more conspicuous.

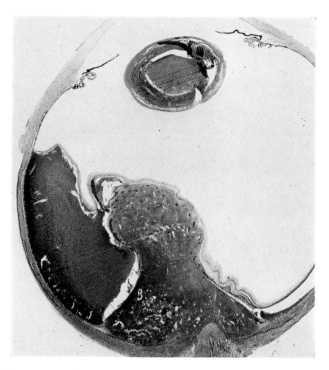

Figure 78. A more advanced choroidal melanoma than that shown in Figure 77, with a typical mushroom shape. The collar of the mushroom is caused by its breaking through the more resistant Bruch's membrane. The head of the mushroom is the tumor growing in the subretinal space. The retina is still adherent to the peak of the tumor but shows an extensive detachment over one slope. The head of the tumor shows numerous enlarged blood vessels.

Reel XIII-5. Regressed retinoblastoma

The left fundus of a 5½-year-old girl. The mother of this patient had an eye removed as a child because of retinoblastoma. Her younger sister had bilateral retinoblastoma and was treated with x-radiation and chemotherapy.

The patient under discussion here had only one lesion in the left eye which regressed from an active tumor into this atrophic scar. The retina is still elevated on the right side of the photograph and is opaque in this area. On the left, the retina is pigmented. Beneath it is an area of choroidal atrophy. This is, therefore, one of the rare cases of hereditary retinoblastoma which regressed spontaneously.

Reel XIII-6. Retinal hemangioma

The right eye of a 13-year-old boy. The left eye was entirely normal. Vision in both eyes was 6/6. The findings in the temporal and lower quandrant of the right fundus were incidental to an examination for a refractive error.

In this segment of the fundus there is a small collection of tortuous, thick blood vessels. They are coiled up, forming a definite tumor. This group of blood vessels has a little gray band in the center. Around this group of

111

Text continued on p. 116.

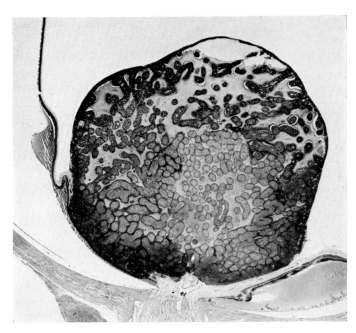

Figure 79. A small retinoblastoma arising from the retina and lying over the optic nerve head. This type of growth which primarily extends into the vitreous cavity is called the "endophytic" type.

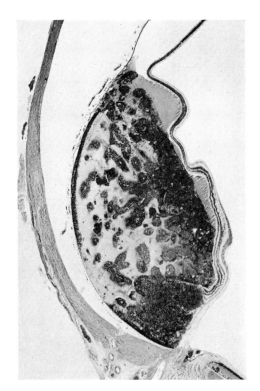

Figure 80. The other type of growth of a retinoblastoma, namely, toward the subretinal space. Here the bulk of the tumor lies between the choroid and the retina. This is the so-called "exophytic" type of growth.

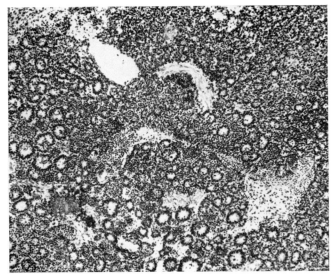

Fig. 81

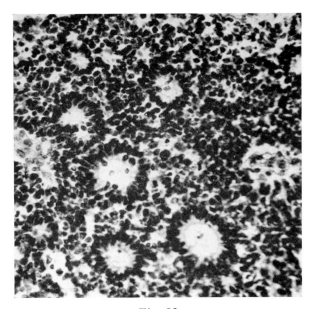

Fig. 82

Figures 81 and 82. Some of the characteristics of a retinoblastoma under high magnification. These are the rosettes which show tumor cells arranged around a lumen. Necrotic areas can also be seen, and these are frequently calcified. Such a rapidly growing tumor easily outgrows its blood supply.

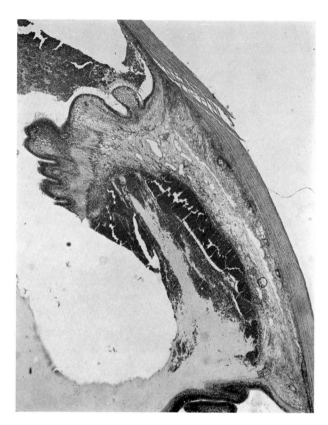

Figure 83. A peripheral retinal hemangioma found in a child whose eye was enucleated because of a peripheral, solid, retinal detachment. In the periphery of this retina was found an accumulation of dilated and new-formed blood vessels. They have produced a retinal fold and a massive hemorrhage.

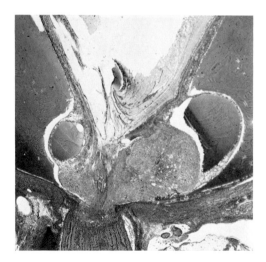

Figure 84. The enucleation was done because a retinoblastoma was suspected in this child. An angiomatous tumor was found near the optic nerve head, which has led to a complete retinal detachment. The tumor itself consists of endothelial cells, capillaries, and vascular proliferation. This is then a so-called hemangioblastoma of the retina (Von Hippel's disease).

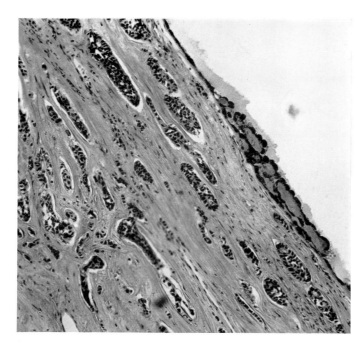

Figure 85. Choroid densely infiltrated with a scirrhous carcioma from the breast. The pigment epithelium can be seen at the upper border of the photomicrograph. The retina has been artifactitiously detached. Breast cancer is the most frequent tumor metastasizing to the choroid. It is frequently a late complication of breast cancer.

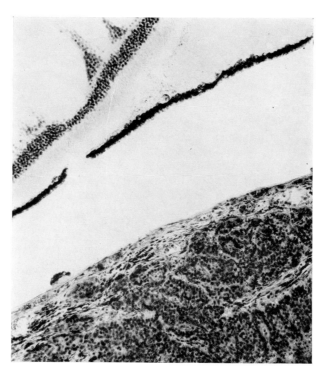

Figure 86. Choroid thickly infiltrated with an adenocarcinoma coming from the intestinal tract. The pigment epithelium above it has been artifactitiously detached. The retina shows large cystoid spaces.

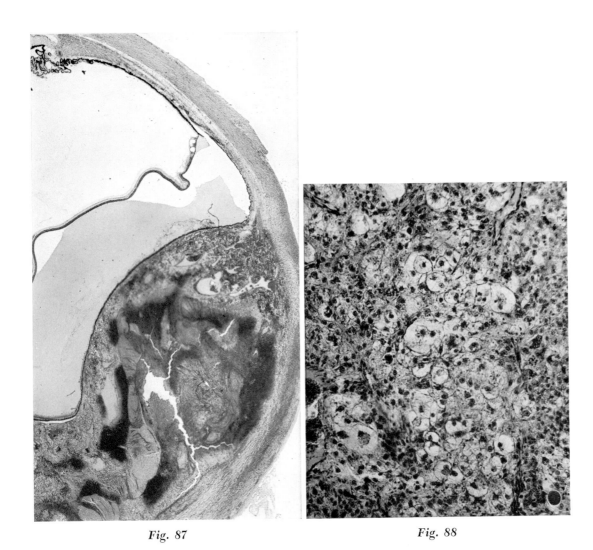

Fig. 87   Fig. 88

Figures 87 and 88. Metastatic hypernephroma. The low magnification (Figure 87) shows the extensive tumor within the choroid, causing a considerable retinal detachment. The high magnification (Figure 88) shows the characteristic cells of this tumor. This eye was enucleated because the clinical picture simulated a choroidal melanoma. Only the histologic examination of the globe revealed the true nature of the lesion, and only then could the tumor of the kidney be detected.

blood vessels a few small red spots can be seen which also could be a small vascular dilatation.

Such vascular anomalies in the periphery of the fundus are frequently the forerunner of so-called Coats' disease. It is assumed that these dilated and thin-walled vessels start to leak into the retinal tissues, causing retinal edema and hemorrhage. In addition, there will soon follow exudation under the retina, with retinal detachment. The end result is a hemorrhagic retinal detachment with numerous yellowish exudates and dilated blood vessels in the retina itself. When such lesions are detected early, light coagulation may be indicated.

Note: The astigmatic "smearing" of the image is due to the extreme angle of view through the optics of the eye.

116

Reel XIII-7. Metastatic tumor of choroid

The left fundus of a 75-year-old white man. The patient suffered from painless loss of vision for three months before he came to our clinic, and a bronchogenic carcinoma had been diagnosed six months before we saw him.

The left fundus shows an elevated grayish-yellow tumor. The lesion lies certainly beneath the retina but has caused a retinal detachment in the macular area. The center of the lesion appears reddish, while the periphery has a yellowish-white, solid character. The retina itself seems edematous but is otherwise unaffected.

Note: The bright orange color at the left, seen with the left eye, is a photographic artifact due to prismatic separation of light in the eye.

Retinal detachment
and
light coagulation

Reel XIV-1. Retinal detachment

The left eye of a 62-year-old white woman. The patient lost the vision in her left eye three weeks before she came to our clinic with a left retinal detachment. Vision in that eye was reduced to hand movements at 1 foot. The right eye showed only a posterior vitreous detachment, and vision in that eye was 6/12.

The photograph of the left fundus gives an overall picture of the detached upper retina. The camera was focused on the balloonlike, elevated part of the retina. The lower retina and the disc can be seen, out of focus, behind the detached retina. The surface of the detached retina shows the fine ripples and folds so characteristic for a serous detachment.

A large horseshoe tear was found in the periphery at the 12 o'clock meridian. A scleral buckling operation with encircling silicone sleeve was performed. The postoperative course was uneventful.

Reel XIV-2. Retinal tear

The right eye of a 60-year-old woman. The patient had had a cataract extraction in both eyes three years previously. Two weeks before she came to us, she noticed a rather sudden loss of vision in the left eye. She noticed a definite defect in the nasal field on that side.

When she was admitted to our clinic, vision in the right eye with correction was 6/6 − 2. The left eye had a large temporal detachment, and vision with correction on that side was 6/21. The right eye showed a flat detachment on the temporal side, with a large horseshoe tear in the 10

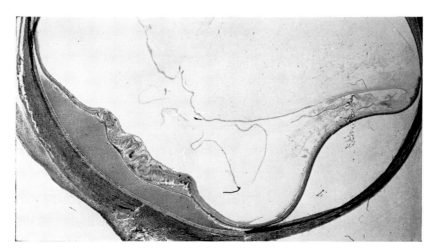

Figure 89. A circumscribed retinal detachment near the posterior pole. The detachment is characterized by the elevation of the retina from the pigment epithelium by a stainable, serous fluid. In addition, the retina is wrinkled and folded. This is clearly visible on the left side of the photomicrograph. In contrast to this, there is an artifactitious retinal detachment on the right side of the photomicrograph in which the subretinal space appears empty and the retina is not folded.

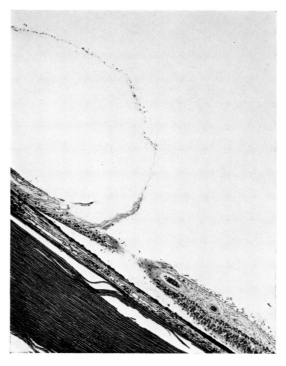

Figure 90. A peripheral retinal hole. There is an interruption of the retina in the center of the photomicrograph. A strand of vitreous remains attached to the anterior lip of this hole.

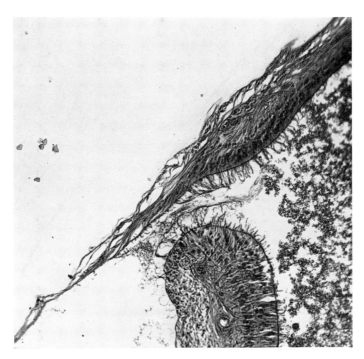

Figure 91. Another cross section through a retinal tear. The posterior lip of the tear, which is in the lower part of the photomicrograph, has a characteristic rounded edge. The anterior lip tapers off into a strand of vitreous which is adherent to this area. The vitreous lies on the left side of the picture, whereas the subretinal fluid is clearly visible on the right side.

o'clock meridian. One week later a scleral buckling procedure, with the implantation of a silicone rod and an encircling tube, was done on the left eye.

The photograph shows, in high magnification, the area of the tear in the right eye. The horseshoelike defect of the retina appears as a dark red area. The apex of this tear points toward the optic nerve head. Between the two branches of the horseshoe, the torn-off retina (operculum) sticks out into the vitreous. A vitreous strand is frequently attached to the tip of such an operculum, the pull of which causes the retina to break.

The right eye was treated with a trapdoor operation and the hole was closed. Vision in that eye remained 6/6.

Reel XIV-3. Retinal hole (photocoagulated)

The left eye of a 61-year-old white woman. Thirteen months before the patient came to our clinic, she had an uncomplicated cataract extraction on the left eye. Three weeks before admission she noticed colored stars, dark spots, and, finally, a lacy curtain over the left eye. A retinal detachment was diagnosed, and a retinal tear was seen in the 11 o'clock meridian. A trapdoor scleral resection was done and a silicone sleeve implanted. During the postoperative examination it was found that the tear was on the buckle, but its posterior end was very close to the posterior slope of the buckle. Five days later the retinal tear was treated with light coagulation.

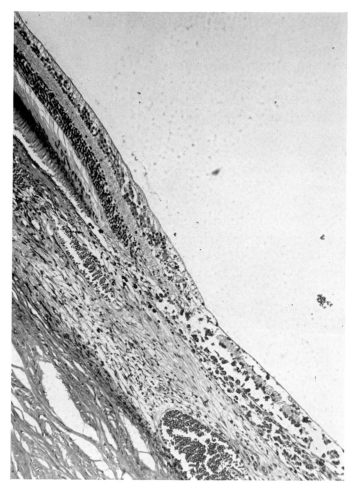

Figure 92. An area of the retina which was treated with light coagulation. A conspicuous chorioretinal scar is present. The retina is necrotic, and the choroid is replaced by connective tissue. There is, however, a dense adhesion between these two layers, and this is the goal for which one usually aims.

After that procedure, the vision returned to 6/9 with aphakic correction. However, in the following months a few vitreous opacities developed, and traction folds were visible in the macular area. Because of these macular changes, the vision slowly decreased to 6/60.

Six months later there was again a questionable elevation of the retina in the area of the original hole. Therefore, this area was again treated with photocoagulation. The photograph was taken one month after this second treatment. Vision at that time with correction was 6/30. The reaction to the photocoagulation was satisfactory. Later on, the patient had an uncomplicated cataract extraction in the right eye and could be observed for another year. The left eye did not change materially, and vision in that eye remained around 6/21.

The photograph shows, under high magnification, the retinal periphery and the hole in the left eye. The hole is still visible as a somewhat collapsed horseshoe. It is surrounded by pigmentation and atrophic scars. The retina in this area seems elevated and edematous.

Reel XIV-4. Retinal hole on scleral buckle

The left eye of a 51-year-old white man. A few days before admission to our clinic, the patient experienced some blurriness of vision in the left eye. When he came to us, vision in the right eye was 6/6, and this eye was essentially normal. Vision in the left eye was 6/6 — 2, and a flat detachment was noticed in the temporal, outer quadrant. The patient was aphakic in both eyes, a cataract extraction having been done about two years previously.

Three small holes were found in the retina, two in the 3 o'clock meridian and one in the 4 o'clock meridian. The patient was put on bedrest for about two weeks, and then a scleral buckling procedure was done under general anesthesia. An encircling silicone tape was placed around the eye. Beneath the tape a silicone implant was put over the area of scleral resection. The scleral tape was tightened to elevate the buckle. As the ocular pressure increased, urea was injected intravenously. The holes were found to be on the buckle.

Since the diathermy reaction around the holes was not sufficient, the holes three days later were surrounded by light coagulations. This was repeated four weeks later when this photograph was taken.

The picture shows the periphery of the left eye with the highly elevated buckle. At the edge of the buckle in the center of the photograph is an area of pigmentation which was caused by the light coagulation of a small retinal hole.

Reels XIV-5, XIV-6, and XIV-7. Retinal telangiectasia (before and after photocoagulation)

The right eye of a 60-year-old white woman. The patient came to our clinic because of a decrease of vision in the right eye. At that time, visual acuity in the right eye was reduced to counting fingers at 2 feet. The right eye showed a dense vitreous hemorrhage, and the right fundus could not be seen. The left eye was essentially normal. The patient returnd one month later, and vision in the right eye had improved remarkably to 6/9 — 2. The fundus could be seen, and it was apparent that the blood had come from a small branch of the inferior temporal artery. It was thought that the hemorrhage was due to her hypertensive cardiovascular disease.

Six months later she had another vitreous hemorrhage in the right eye. Vision was reduced to 6/21. At that time there was also a hemorrhage visible in the retina near the macular area. Her hypertension was brought under control. The patient did not have any signs of diabetes.

When she returned one month later, the vitreous hemorrhage again had cleared. Vision was improved to 6/9, and areas of newly formed blood vessels were seen at the posterior pole above and temporal to the macula. These newly formed blood vessels were thought to be either small retinal hemangiomas or telangiectasias. Since they were the source of repeated bleedings, light coagulation was done.

The first photograph (Reel XIV-5) shows the area of the most pronounced neovascularization above the right macula one day before light coagulation was applied. Clusters of new-formed blood vessels can be seen sprouting out from the upper temporal artery. They form loops and angioma-like nodules.

The second photograph (Reel XIV-6) shows the same area two days after the application of light coagulation. The areas of coagulation in the pigment epithelium and choroid are plainly visible as yellowish-white foci. The main artery seems to be attenuated and carries less blood. The angioma-like blood vessels are less numerous and less pronounced.

The third photograph (Reel XIV-7) shows the same area one month after light coagulation. Practically all of the newly formed blood vessels have disappeared. In the deeper parts of the retina and in the choroid lies a partly pigmented, partly atrophic scar. Only a few superficial hemorrhages and the shadows of former blood vessels remain of the original lesion. The main artery is somewhat thin but carries blood.

The patient was observed for two more years, and she did not experience any more vitreous hemorrhages in this eye.

Vitreous and
trauma

Reel XV-1. Vitreous opacities

The right eye of a 37-year-old white man. This patient had numerous congenital anomalies. He had an arteriovenous aneurysm of the middle cerebral vessels due to an angiomatous-like malformation. This was resected three years before we saw him. Also, in the past he had had numerous attacks of very severe headaches accompanied by vomiting and blurring of vision. Occasionally he would become unconscious. These attacks became more prominent before the craniotomy was performed. He had periods where he remained comatose for up to ten to fourteen days. He finally was left with a right hemiparesis, a right hemianopsia, and a profound expressive dysphasia. After the operation, the patient improved considerably. The dysphasia and hemiparesis disappeared. The hemianopsia, however, remained. He still suffered from occasional convulsions.

Vision in the right eye was 6/6, and the only anomaly noticed in this eye was this striking vitreous opacity. It is weblike and thin. It consists of a somewhat denser but yet transparent core from which several strands extend into the periphery. The fundus can be seen through this opacity.

This is a good example of a conspicuous vitreous opacity as it occurs occasionally after an intraocular inflammation or as a degenerative phenomenon in patients with senile vitreous changes or with high myopia. In this patient, however, we must assume that this was a congenital anomaly since no inflammation preceded the vitreous opacity.

Vision in the left eye was reduced to 6/21. The macula showed pigmentary changes, and the retinal vessels on this side showed a marked

124

tortuosity and dilatation. There was also an indication of new formation of retinal blood vessels.

In addition to this congenital vitreous opacity in the right eye, the patient suffers from vascular anomalies of the retina and the brain. This entity has been grouped with other diffuse hamartomatoses or so-called phakomatoses. It was fully described by Wyburn-Mason.*

Reel XV-2. Asteroid hyalitis

The left eye of an 85-year-old white woman. The patient came to our clinic for a refraction. Vision in both eyes could be corrected to 6/9, and there was no other ocular pathologic finding.

The photograph shows the vitreous opacities against the red fundus. These opacities have been compared to snowballs or stars on a clear night. The opacities are suspended in the vitreous and move with the vitreous but do not settle down as do the crystals in synchysis scintillans. These opacities usually do not interfere with vision, but they may become so dense that visual acuity is reduced. Recent histopathologic and histochemical observations† have suggested that these lipid bodies arise from some type of degeneration of the vitreous fibrils.

Reel XV-3. Retinal vessels elevated toward vitreous

The left eye of a 55-year-old white housewife. The patient had never seen well with her left eye. The eye had never caused any real trouble, but she has always been concerned about the poor vision in that eye. The right eye was normal, and vision in that eye with correction was 6/15.

When the patient came to our clinic, vision in the left eye was reduced to doubtful light perception. The left eye was in a divergent position with an exotropia of about 10°. There was also a slight left hypertropia. The right visual field was normal, and the left visual field showed a large central scotoma. The left fundus showed an oblique optic nerve head with a supertraction of the retina on the nasal and superior margin. The retina appeared thinner at the posterior pole.

Above and below the macula, extending temporally into the periphery, are discrete clumps of pigment. Below this pigmentation is a highly elevated, gray, horizontal fold of the superficial part of the retina which carries the retinal vessels in it.

Reel XV-4. Deep peripapillary hemorrhage

The left fundus of an 83-year-old white woman. Vision in the right eye had been reduced for more than a year, but the patient always had good

---

*Wyburn-Mason, R.: Arteriovenous aneurysm of midbrain and retina, facial nevi and mental changes, Brain 66:163-203, 1943.

†Rodman, H. I., Johnson, F. B., and Zimmerman, L. E.: New histopathological and histochemical observations concerning asteroid hyalitis, Arch. Ophth. 66:552-563, 1961.

125

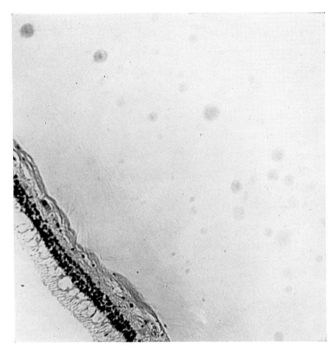

Fig. 93

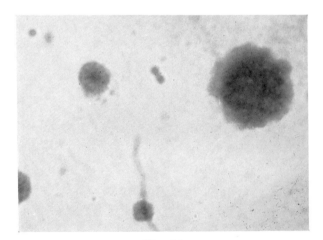

Fig. 94

Figures 93 and 94. The vitreous opacities of asteroid hyalitis are seen on the histologic section as faintly staining deposits in the vitreous near the retinal surface. They are of different size and density. Most of them appear round or slightly oval. In high magnification (Figure 94) they can be seen suspended in the vitreous meshwork.

vision in the left eye. A few days before she came to us, she noticed sudden loss of vision in the left eye after a trivial trauma.

The right eye showed an almost mature cortical senile cataract, and vision in that eye was reduced to light perception and correct projection. In the left eye vision was reduced to counting fingers at 2 feet. The left lens showed only a few peripheral spokes. In the left fundus is a dense, dark bluish, raised lesion which is temporal to the disc margin. It extends to and beyond the macula. The retinal vessels can be seen crossing over this lesion, and they are slightly elevated.

The hemorrhage cleared very slowly, with partial restoration of vision.

Reel XV-5. Papilledema with traumatic cerebral edema

The left eye of a 9-year-old boy. Two weeks before this photograph was taken, the child fell from a fourteen-foot wall. He fell on concrete, and broke one arm. He was not unconscious but complained of blurred vision after the accident. He also complained of headaches off and on.

When the patient was seen by us, vision in both eyes was 6/9. The anterior segments were normal in both eyes. There was a papilledema of 4-diopter elevation on both sides.

The photograph of the left fundus shows the highly elevated nerve head. Its margin is blurred, and there is some whitish exudation at the lower rim. The veins are somewhat dilated. Deep yellowish retinal depos-

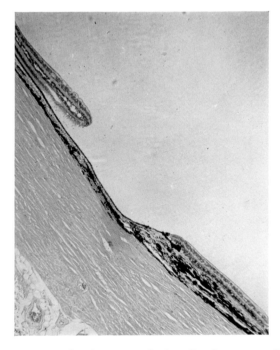

Figure 95. Posterior pole of an eye which suffered a severe, blunt trauma. The retina is interrupted in the macular area and shows a large macular hole. On one side is a hypertrophic scar with marked pigmentation. This corresponded clinically to an indirect choroidal rupture. On the left side the macular hole has a blunt edge characteristic of such a lesion. The retina in this area shows cystoid degeneration.

127

its are visible around the disc, especially on the temporal side toward the macula. There, they are forming an incomplete star figure.

The neurologic examination revealed only a slightly increased pressure in the cerebrospinal fluid. All of the other examinations remained negative, and the boy recovered within four weeks.

Reel XV-6. Traumatic chorioretinal atrophy

The right fundus of a 38-year-old white man. One day before the patient came to our clinic, he was hammering on a U joint. Some foreign body hit his right eye, and he had blurred vision since then.

When we saw him, he had a linear perforation of the right cornea and a small iris hole in the 2 o-clock meridian. The lens showed beginning opacities in the upper, outer quadrant. The retina was edematous, and with the ophthalmoscope a small foreign body could be seen below the macula. Vision in the right eye was reduced to 6/12. The left eye was and has remained normal. On the same day, the foreign body was extracted with the hand magnet.

Below the macula in the area where the foreign body had been lodged, a pigmented scar developed. This, however, did not interfere with vision, and since the cataract did not progress, visual acuity returned to 6/6.

In this area of chorioretinal atrophy there is a great deal of pigment dissemination. The black pigment lies superficially as well as deep in the retina. The choroid underneath it shows a patchy atrophy. This lesion was probably caused by the impact of the metallic foreign body.

Reel XV-7. Indirect choroidal rupture

The right eye of a 43-year-old white machinist. The patient's right eye had been injured twenty-five years previously when a hard, blunt object was thown against him. He lost central vision immediately in this eye but has had no further difficulties.

When he was seen by us, vision in the right eye was reduced to 6/60 eccentrically. The right anterior segment was normal. The right fundus shows a protruding jet-black mass in the macular area. This mass lies in the retina itself but is surrounded by some less dense pigmentation in the deeper layers. From this pigment mass goes a curvilinear scar downward and nasally. This scar appears as a white ribbon in which there are a few pigment dots. It lies deep to the retina, and the retinal vessels cross over it. Only part of this scar is visible on the photograph. It extended farther down and nasally, lying circumferentially to the disc. The left eye was entirely normal, and vision in that eye was 6/5.

Index

130